Recent Results in Cancer Research 134

Managing Editors
Ch. Herfarth, Heidelberg · H.-J. Senn, St. Gallen

Associate Editors
M. Baum, London · V. Diehl, Köln
F. Gutzwiller, Zürich · M.F. Rajewsky, Essen
M. Wannenmacher, Heidelberg

Founding Editor
P. Rentchnick, Geneva

H.-D. Pape U. Ganzer
G. Schmitt (Eds.)

Carcinoma of the Oral Cavity and Oropharynx

With 43 Figures and 52 Tables

Springer-Verlag
Berlin Heidelberg New York
London Paris Tokyo
Hong Kong Barcelona
Budapest

Prof. Dr. med. Dr. med. dent. H.-D. Pape
Klinik und Poliklinik für Zahn-, Mund- und Kieferheilkunde, Mund-, Kiefer- und Gesichtschirurgie
Joseph-Stelzmann-Str. 9
50931 Köln
Germany

Prof. Dr. med. U. Ganzer
Hals-, Nasen- und Ohrenklinik
Universität Düsseldorf
Moorenstr. 5
40225 Düsseldorf
Germany

Prof. Dr. med. G. Schmitt
Klinik für Strahlentherapie
Universität Düsseldorf
Moorenstr. 5
40225 Düsseldorf
Germany

ISBN 3-540-56819-0 Springer-Verlag Berlin Heidelberg New York
ISBN 0-387-56819-0 Springer-Verlag New York Berlin Heidelberg

CIP data applied for

Typesetting: Best-set Typesetter Ltd., Hong Kong
19/3130/SPS-5 4 3 2 1 0 – Printed on acid-free paper

Invited Speakers and Chairmen

Beck, L., Prof. Dr.
Universitäts Frauenklinik, Moorenstr. 5, D-40225, Düsseldorf, Germany

Bier, H., PD Dr.
Heinrich-Heine-Universität Düsseldorf, Hals-Nasen-Ohrenklinik, Moorenstr. 5, D-40225 Düsseldorf, Germany

Bier, J., Prof. Dr. Dr.
Universitätsklinikum Rudolf Virchow, Abt. für Mund-, Kiefer- und Gesichtschirurgie und Plastische Operationen, Augustenburger Platz 1, D-13353 Berlin, Germany

Biörklund, A., Prof. M.D.
University Hospital of Lund, Department of Oto-Rhino-Laryngology, S-221 85 Lund, Sweden

Boysen, M., Prof. Dr.
University of Oslo, Dept. of Otolaryngology, Rikshospitalet, N-0027 Oslo 1/Norway

Carlson, E.R., D.M.D.
Henry Ford Hospital, Oral and Maxillofacial Surgery, Dept. of Surgery, 2799 West Grand Boulevard, Detroit, MI 48202, USA

Donald, P.J., M.D., F.R.C.S.(C)
University of California, Dept. of Otolaryngology, 2500 Stockton Blvd., Sacramento, CA 95817, USA

Duncan, G.F., M.S.
Graphica Sculptura Medica, P.O. Box 446, Rochester, MN 55903, USA

Eschwège, F., Prof. Dr.
Service de Radiothérapie, Institute Gustave Roussy, Rue Camille Desmoulin, F-94805 Villejuif, France

Fu, Karen K., M.D.
Dept. of Radiat. Oncology, University of San Francisco (U.C.S.F.), San Francisco, CA, USA

Ganzer, U., Prof. Dr.
Heinrich-Heine-Universität Düsseldorf, Hals-Nasen-Ohrenklinik, Moorenstr. 5 D-40225 Düsseldorf, Germany

Hausamen, J.-E., Prof. Dr. Dr.
Medizinische Hochschule Hannover, Abt. für Mund-, Kiefer- und Gesichtschirurgie, Postfach 61 01 80
D-30623 Hannover, Germany

Horiot, J.C. Prof. M.D.
Centre Georges-Francois-Leclerc, Unité de Radiothérapie, 1, Rue du Professeur Marion, 1, F-21034 Dijon, Cedex, France

Howaldt, H.P., PD Dr. Dr.
Johann Wolfgang Goethe Universität, Abt. für Mund-, Kiefer u. Gesichtschirurgie, Theodor-Stern-Kai 7,
D-60596 Frankfurt, Germany

von Ilberg, C., Prof. Dr.
Johann Wolfgang Goethe-Universität, Hals-Nasen-Ohrenklinik, Theodor-Stern-Kai 7, D-60596 Frankfurt, Germany

Mazeron, J.-J., M.D.
Hopital Henri Mondor, 51 Avenue du Maréchal, de Lattre de Tassigny, F-94010 Créteil, France

Mohr, Ch., Prof. Dr. Dr.
Universitätsklinikum Essen, Klinik f. Gesichts- und Kieferchirurgie, Hufelandstr. 55, D-45147 Essen, Germany

Müller, R.P. Prof. Dr.
Klinik u. Poliklinik, für Strahlentherapie der Universität zu Köln, Joseph-Stelzmann Str. 9, D-50931 Köln, Germany

Pape, H.-D. Prof. Dr. Dr.
Abt. für Mund-, Kiefer- und Gesichtschirurgie der Universität zu Köln, Joseph-Stelzmann Str. 9, D-50931 Köln, Germany

Parsons, J.T., M.D.
University of Florida, Dept. of Radiation Oncology, PO Box 100385, Gainesville, FL 32610-0385, USA

Pindborg, J.J., Prof. D.M.D.
Royal Dental College, Dept. of Oral Pathology, 20 Norre Allé, DK-2200 Copenhagen N, Denmark

Schmidt-Ullrich, R., M.D.
Medical College of Virginia Hospitals, Dept. of Radiation Oncology, Clinical Section, Box 58-MCV Station, Richmond, VA 23298-0058, USA

Schmitt, G., Prof. Dr.
Heinrich-Heine-Universität Düsseldorf, Strahlentherapeutische Klinik, Moorenstr. 5, D-40225 Düsseldorf, Germany

Schnabel, Th., Dr.
Heinrich-Heine-Universität Düsseldorf, Strahlentherapeutische Klinik, Moorenstr. 5, D-40225 Düsseldorf, Germany

Snow, G.B. Prof. Dr.
Free University Hospital, Dept. of Oto-Rhino-Laryngology, Head and Neck Surgery, De Boelelaan 1117, NL-1081 HV Amsterdam, The Netherlands

de Vries N., Dr.
Free University Hospital, Dept. of Oto-Rhino-Laryngology, Head and Neck Surgery, De Boelelaan 1117, NL-1081 HV Amsterdam, The Netherlands

Wolf, G.T., Prof. M.D.
University of Michigan, Dept. of Otolaryngology, 1904 Taubman Center, 1500 E. Medical Center Drive, Ann Arbor, MI 48109, USA

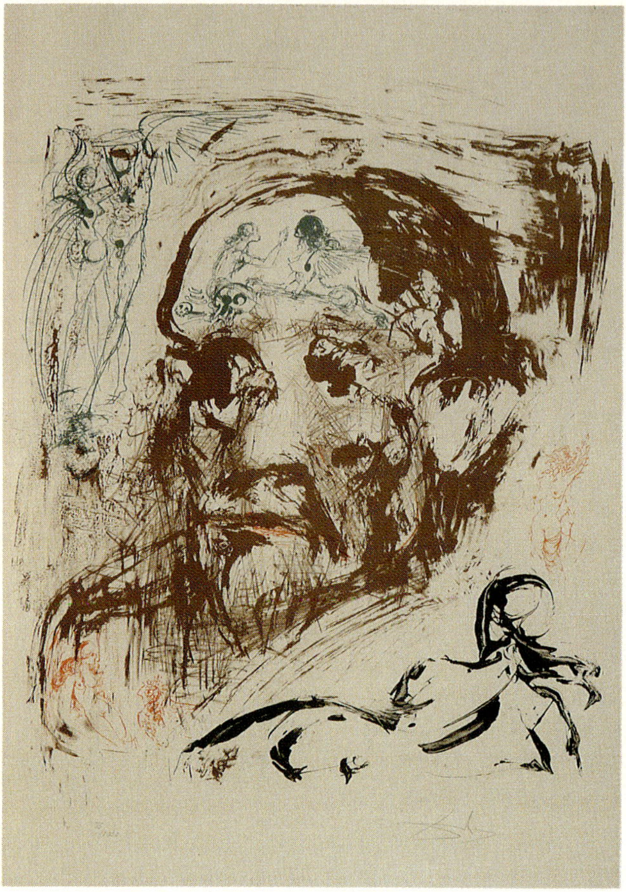

The fate of Sigmund Freud, born in 1856 in Vienna, is typical of the fate of patients with carcinoma of the oral mucosa. He smoked up to 20 cigars a day during his adult life. In 1923, a leukoplakial carcinoma of the right arcus palatopharyngeus was diagnosed. There followed 16 years of suffering with repeated relapses and increasing deformation of the surrounding tissue structures. The maxillofacial surgeon Pichler, who treated him up to his death in 1939, records 12 operations and the repeated use of radium therapy. This drawing by Dali shows him shortly before his death.

Preface

A 40% chance of survival is generally attributed to patients with cancer of the oral mucosa and of the oropharynx. The rate has remained constant over the past three decades, despite the medical progress thus far achieved. There are two reasons for this.

Firstly, it has to be noted that since 70% of tumors treated for the first time have a diameter greater than 2 cm, therapy is obviously begun too late in most cases. In addition, carcinomas of this kind have been continually increasing not only in relative, but also in absolute numbers. Epidemiological data show that this alarming trend has manifested itself over the past decades: in the FRG in the 1960s, three men and one women per 100 000 inhabitants could be expected to develop this form of cancer. To date, the rate has doubled, although it is interesting that among the whole spectrum of cancers, the percentage of carcinomas of the oral mucosa and oropharynx is much lower in Germany than in other countries. Certain unhealthy habits are responsible for the increase observed in Germany, such as smoking and excessive alcohol consumption. Therefore, the early detection of precancerous and malignant lesions as well as preventive measures are acquiring significant importance in the management of cancers of the oral cavity and oropharynx.

Secondly, even by combining surgery, radiotherapy, and antineoplastic chemotherapy, we have not been able to substantially improve the survival rate in patients with advanced disease. In these three disciplines, each with their different priorities, sharing recent experience and ideas is of the utmost importance.

The surgical treatment of carcinomas of the head and neck has made great progress over the past 20 years, particularly as a result of the opportunities opened up by tissue replacement. Nevertheless, even increasingly radical surgery has failed to really improve the chances of survival. Only the carefully organized combination of surgery, radiotherapy, and chemotherapy seems promising as far as improvement using less invasive surgery and eventually achieving better quality of life are concerned.

We hope that this book will contribute to the process. European and American experts from the three disciplines involved – ear, nose, and throat (ENT), maxilofacial surgery (MFS), and radiotherapy (RT) – have surveyed the current status of knowledge and the treatment perspectives for the years to come, extensive clinical experience being the basis of the contributions.

The particular advantage of international organizations for the documentation of tumors as well as for the inauguration of larger therapy studies has been shown by the presentations made by the German, Austrian, and Swiss Association for Head and Neck Tumors (DÖSAK) and the European Organization for Research on Treatment of Cancer (EORTC). It is in these associations that important steps are being taken in the joint care of patients, and it is here, too, that one may expect to find objective and realistic data to evaluate these forms of cancer. If the chance of survival can be improved, the requirements for aftercare and rehabilitation will also increase and become more distinct. Reconstructions and functional restoration in the head and neck region and a better quality of life for individual patients are the objectives common to all the articles in this volume.

Köln H.-D. Pape
December 1993

Contents

A. Biörklund and J. Wennersberg
Epidemiology of Cancer of the Oral Cavity and Oropharynx 1

J.J. Pindborg
Clinical Relevance of Precancerous Lesions of Oral Mucosa 9

P.J. Donald
Extended Surgery for Advanced Maxillary Sinus Carcinoma 17

J.-E. Hausamen and F.W. Neukam
Resection of Tumors in Tongue, Floor of the Mouth, and Mandible: Possibilities of Primary Reconstruction 25

C. von Ilberg
Surgery of Oropharyngeal Cancer 37

G.B. Snow, M.W.M. van den Brekel, C.R. Leemans, and P. Patel
Surgical Management of Cervical Lymph Nodes in Patients with Oral and Oropharyngeal Cancer 43

J. Bier
Radical Neck Dissection Versus Conservative Neck Dissection for Squamous Cell Carcinoma of the Oral Cavity 57

F. Eschwège, P. Wibault, A. Lusinchi, A. Gerbaulet, P. Marandas, C. Domenge, and B. Luboinski
Treatment of Oropharynx Carcinomas: Experience at the Institut Gustave-Roussy 63

R.K. Schmidt-Ullrich, C.R. Johnson, S. Khandelwal, and D.E. Wazer
Concomitant Boost-Accelerated, Superfractionated Irradiation for the Treatment of Advanced Carcinomas of the Oral Cavity and Oropharynx 69

J.T. Parsons, R.R. Million, and W.M. Mendenhall
Regional Lymph Node Irradiation 81

T. Schnabel, N. Zamboglou, H. Bier, C.U. Fritzemeier, H. Bojar, E.T. Merholz, C. Kolotas, and G. Schmitt
Radiotherapy with Different Fractionations and Simultaneous Cisplatin or Carboplatin in the Treatment of Advanced Head and Neck Carcinomas: Clinical Results and Radiobiological Investigations 89

J.-J. Mazeron, L. Grimard, and V. Benk
Curietherapy Versus External Irradiation Combined with Curietherapy in Stage II Squamous Cell Carcinomas of Mobile Tongue and Floor of the Mouth 101

J.C. Horiot, A.C. Begg, R. Le Fur, S. Schraub, W. van den Bogaert, M. van Glabbeke, and M. Pierart
Present Status of EORTC Trials of Hyperfractionated and Accelerated Radiotherapy on Head and Neck Carcinoma 111

N. de Vries
Second Primary Tumors in Oral and Oropharyngeal Cancer 121

G.T. Wolf, S. Urba, and M. Hazuka
Induction Chemotherapy for Organ Preservation in Advanced Squamous Cell Carcinoma of the Oral Cavity and Oropharynx 133

K.K. Fu, J.D. Cox, T.F. Pajak, V.A. Marcial, L.R. Coia, M. Mohiuddin, H.M. Selim, R.W. Byhardt, S. McDonald, H.G. Ortiz, and L. Martin

Carcinomas of the Oropharynx Treated with Hyperfractionated Radiation Therapy on Radiation Therapy Oncology Group Protocol 8313 145

C. Mohr, W. Bohndorf, H. Gremmel, F. Härle, J.-E. Hausamen, H. Hirche, M. Molls, K.H. Renner, J. Reuther, H. Sack, D. Schettler, H. Scheunemann, and M. Thelen
Preoperative Radiochemotherapy and Radical Surgery of Advanced Head and Neck Cancers – Results of a Prospective, Multicenter DÖSAK Study 155

R.-P. Müller, S. Staar, M. Samek, and H.-D. Pape
Simultaneous Preoperative Radiochemotherapy with Cisplatin in Advanced Oral Cavity Carcinomas: Acute Response and Follow-Up 165

H.-P. Howaldt, M. Frenz, and H. Pitz
Results from DÖSAK Observational Studies 173

H. Bier
Current Trends in Therapeutic Research 183

E.R. Carlson
The Radiobiology, Treatment, and Prevention of Osteoradionecrosis of the Mandible 191

G.F. Duncan
Epiprosthetic Rehabilitation: Patient's Acceptance of a Facial Epithesis Following Tumor Surgery 201

M. Boysen
Value of Follow-Up in Patients Treated for Squamous Cell Carcinomas of the Oral Cavity and Oropharynx . . 205

Subject Index 215

*List of Contributors**

Begg, A.C. *101*[1]
Benk, V. *101*
Bier, H. *89*, *183*
Bier, J. *57*
Biörklund, A. *1*
Bohndorf, W. *155*
Bojar, H. *89*
Boysen, M. *205*
Byhardt, R.W. *145*
Carlson, E.R. *191*
Coia, L.R. *145*
Cox, J.D. *145*
de Vries, N. *121*
Domenge, C. *63*
Donald, P.J. *17*
Duncan, G.F. *201*
Eschwège, F. *63*
Frenz, M. *173*
Fritzemeier, C.U. *89*
Fu, K.K. *145*
Gerbaulet, A. *63*
Gremmel, H. *155*
Grimard, L. *101*
Härle, F. *155*
Hausamen, J.-E. *25*, *155*
Hazuka, M. *133*
Hirche, H. *155*
Horiot, J.C. *111*
Howaldt, H.-P. *173*
Johnson, C.R. *69*
Khandelval, S. *69*
Kolotas, C. *89*
Leemans, C.R. *43*
Le Fur, R. *111*
Luboinski, B. *63*
Lusinchi, A. *63*
Marandas, P. *63*
Marcial, V.A. *145*
Martin, L. *145*
Mazeron, J.-J. *101*
McDonald, S. *145*
Mendenhall, W.M. *81*
Merholz, E.T. *89*
Million, R.R. *81*
Mohiuddin, M. *145*
Mohr, C. *155*
Molls, M. *155*
Müller, R.-P. *165*
Neukam, F.W. *25*
Ortiz, H.G. *145*
Pajak, T.F. *145*
Pape, H.-D. *165*

* The addresses of the authors are given on the first page of each contribution.

[1] Page on which contribution begins.

Parson, J.T. *81*
Patel, P. *43*
Pierart, M. *111*
Pindborg, J.J. *9*
Pitz, H. *173*
Renner, K.H. *155*
Reuther, J. *155*
Sack, H. *155*
Samek, M. *165*
Schettler, D. *155*
Scheunemann, H. *155*
Schmidt-Ulrich, R.K. *69*
Schmitt, G. *89*
Schnabel, T. *89*
Schraub, S. *111*
Selim, H.M. *145*
Snow, G.B. *43*
Staar, S. *165*
Thelen, M. *155*
Urba, S. *133*
van den Bogaert, W. *111*
van den Brekel, M.W.M. *43*
van Glabbeke, M. *111*
von Ilberg, C. *37*
Wazer, D.E. *69*
Wennersberg, J. *1*
Wibault, P. *63*
Wolf, G.T. *133*
Zamboglou, N. *89*

Epidemiology of Cancer of the Oral Cavity and Oropharynx

A. Biörklund and J. Wennersberg

Department of Otorhinolaryngology, University Hospital, S-221 85 Lund, Sweden

At the present time, there are at least three programs in Europe aiming to reduce cancer mortality: the World Health Organization (WHO), the European Community (EC), and the Nordic Cancer Union are trying to reduce cancer mortality by 15% either in patients below 65 years or in all age groups. This aim may be achieved by different means: primary (prevention), secondary (early diagnosis), and tertiary (improved treatment). Among these primary prevention is often considered to have top priority, which anticipates that risk factors can be eliminated. For this purpose, cancer registration is the basis for national programs of cancer control. It gives information about the influence of preventive measures and cure rates.

Early diagnosis is difficult in cancer of the oral cavity and oropharynx due to diffuse symptoms which may be overlooked both by the doctor and the tumor patient. Treatment may reduce cancer mortality, but in some patients may increase the morbidity to a level considered worse than the disease itself (Temple and Burkitt 1991).

Aspects of the epidemiology of cancer of the oral cavity and oropharynx may be described in terms of the geographical distribution of tumors, sex and age characteristics of the patients, and results of treatment from different time periods. These aspects will then be the basis for different types of studies of risk factors in cancer of the oral cavity and oropharynx.

In different reports on statistics of cancer of the head and neck area, it is almost impossible to identify the oral cavity and oropharynx as two separate sites. All sites for malignant tumors from the lip to the hypopharynx are included in all reports. The tumors are grouped together as cancer of the buccal (oral) cavity (mouth) and pharynx, classified in the International Classification of Diseases (ICD) code as −8, −9, and −0, as site numbers 140–149 (Table 1). These sites (140–149) include both squamous cell carcinomas and other types of cancer with different biological behavior, such as salivary gland carcinomas and nasopharyngeal carcinomas. In addition, the

Table 1. Sites in cancer of the buccal (oral) cavity (mouth) and pharynx; oral cancer; ICD code −8, −9, −0

Site number	Site
140	Lip
141	Tongue (including base of tongue)
142	Major salivary glands
143	Gum
144	Floor of mouth
145	Other unspecified parts of mouth
146	Oropharynx
147	Nasopharynx
148	Hypopharynx
149	Pharynx and ill-defined sites in lip, oral cavity, and pharynx

Table 2. Squamous cell carcinomas by site and differentiation (Roland et al. 1992)

Site	Differentiation (%)			Total number of cases (*n*)
	Good	Moderate	Poor	
Mouth	52	35	13	438
Nasopharynx	14	12	74	43
Hypopharynx	31	36	33	376
Oropharynx	34	33	33	272

Table 3. Estimated numbers of new cases of cancer of the mouth/pharynx (140–149) in 1980 (Parkin et al. 1988)

Area (Europe)	Male (*n*)	Female (*n*)
Eastern	12 000	3000
Northern	9 000	5000[a]
Southern	145 000	3000
Western	20 000	4000

[a] The whole population covered by national cancer registration (excluding Ireland), therefore providing the most accurate figures.

differentiation of squamous cell carcinomas may differ within these sites (Table 2), something that has been studied recently by Roland et al. (1992).

However, the only international reports available for this presentation are those related to buccal cavity/pharynx cancers (140–149). The estimated numbers of new cancers in these sites in Europe are shown in Table 3. It must be stressed that the estimates are only a poor substitute for measure-

Table 4. Estimated average annual incidence of buccal cavity and pharynx cancers from 1978 to 1982 per 100000 inhabitants (Jensen et al. 1990)

Country	Sex	Age-group		
		0–44 years	45–64 years	>65 years
France	M	4.0	113.6	139.8
	F	0.5	7.0	10.5
Germany	M	2.0	28.2	38.6
	F	0.5	4.0	7.0
EC	M	2.0	46.7	66.4
	F	0.5	4.0	10.2
Netherlands	M	0.6	13.1	37.5
	F	0.4	3.7	11.6

ments of cancer incidence by population-based cancer registers. It is only in the northern part of Europe (Nordic countries and the United Kingdom) that the whole population is included in national cancer registration, and these figures are, therefore, considered to be more accurate.

The average annual incidence of buccal cavity and pharynx cancer within the European Community has been analyzed by Jensen et al. (1990) (Table 4). This material is also based on estimated incidence. In Sweden, there are

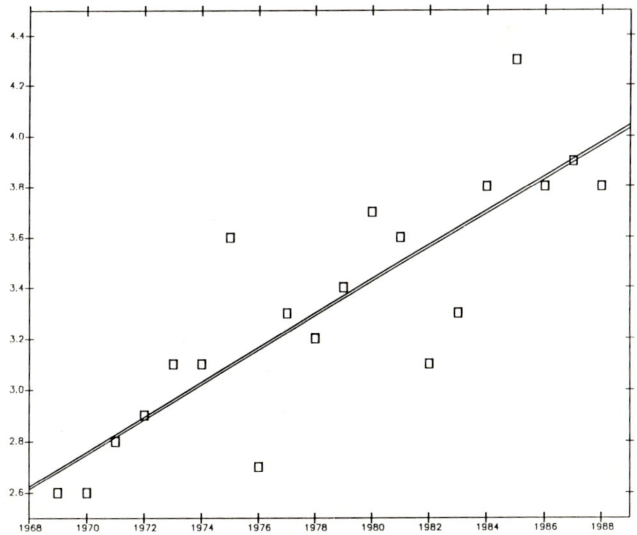

Fig. 1. Cancer of the oral cavity (ICD-9 sites 141, 143–145): age-adjusted rates per 100000 inhabitants in Sweden between 1969 and 1988. *r*, 0.7; *p*, 0.0001

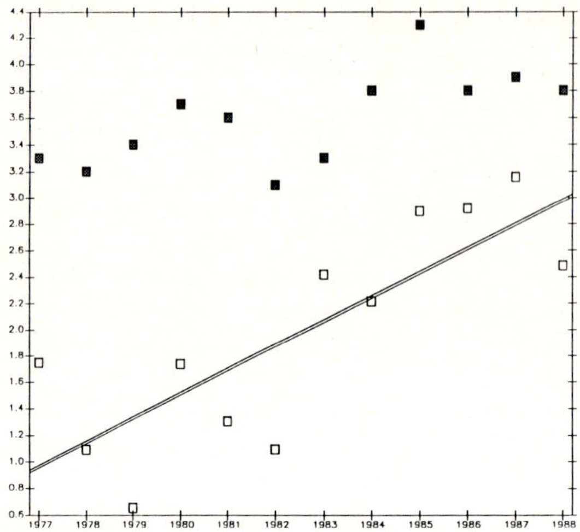

Fig. 2. Cancer of the oral cavity (ICD-9 sites 141, 143–145): age-adjusted rates per 100 000 inhabitants for the whole population (■) and per 1 000 000 for patients younger than 40 years (□) in Sweden between 1977 and 1988. *p*, 0.002

more accurate reports on incidence at different sites. Cancer of the oral cavity and oropharynx can easily be identified as two separate groups and are divided into different subsites in the annual report of the Swedish Cancer Registry (established in 1958). Figures 1 and 2 show data from this registry for cancer of the oral cavity (141 and 143–145, ICD-9), given as age-adjusted rates per 100 000 inhabitants. The rates are from the period 1969–1988, and there is an increase of cancer during this period (National Board of Health and Welfare 1988). In Fig. 2, patients below 40 years of age are represented by age-adjusted rates per 1 million inhabitants. This figure demonstrates a marked rise of the incidence in younger patients compared to the population as a whole. Between 1981 and 1989, a prospective registration was carried out in Sweden of all cancers of the oral cavity (sites 140, 143–145). During this period, 1409 tumor cases were registered, and the stages of these tumors are shown in Table 5. An even distribution of different stages was found. In 73% of all cases, no lymph node metastasis was observed.

Figure 3 shows the incidence rates of cancer of the oropharynx; an increased incidence rate was found during the observation period 1969–1988. Cancer mortality statistics from different time periods are of interest because they may reveal whether therapy has had any influence on the death rate. In Table 6, the age-adjusted death rate for malignant neoplasms of the buccal cavity and pharynx have been registered for France, Germany, and the Netherlands during the three time periods 1952–1953, 1966–1967, and 1984–1985 (Kurihara et al. 1989). The death rate in the Netherlands re-

Table 5. Stages of cancer of the oral cavity (ICD-9, 141, 143–145) from 1981 to 1989 in Sweden

Stage	Distribution (%) (n = 1409)
I	23
II	26
III	21
IV	22
not specified	8

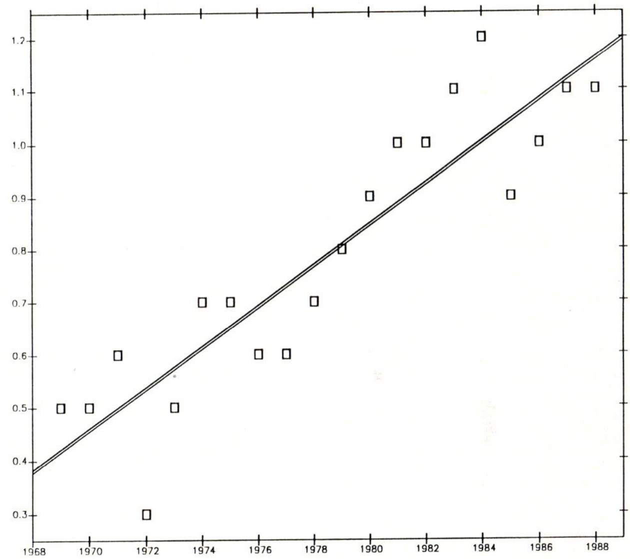

Fig. 3. Cancer of the oropharynx (ICD-9 site 146): age-adjusted rates per 100000 inhabitants in Sweden between 1969 and 1988. r, 0.81; p, 0.0001

Table 6. Age-adjusted death rates for malignant neoplasms of buccal cavity and pharynx (ICD-9 140–149) (Kurihara et al. 1989)

Country	Sex	1952–1953	1966–1976	1984–1985
France	M	5.68	9.96	14.83
	F	0.61	0.79	1.23
Germany, Fed. Rep.	M	1.66	1.80	5.14
	F	0.63	0.51	0.87
Netherlands	M	3.40	2.39	3.87
	F	0.93	0.75	0.77

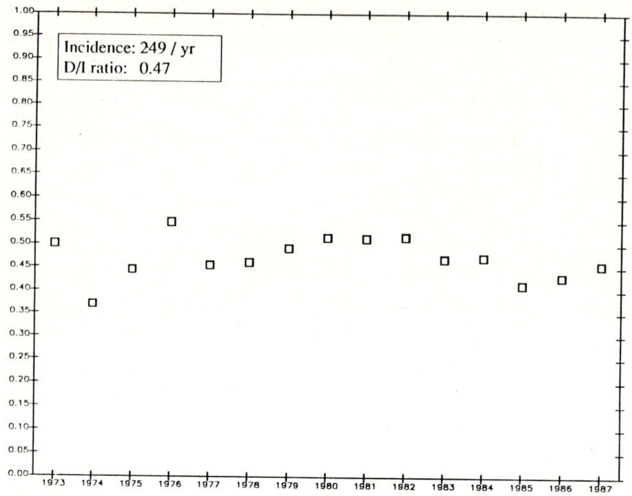

Fig. 4. Cancer of the oral cavity (ICD-9 sites 141, 143–145): number of deaths/new cases (death/incidence) in Sweden between 1973 and 1987

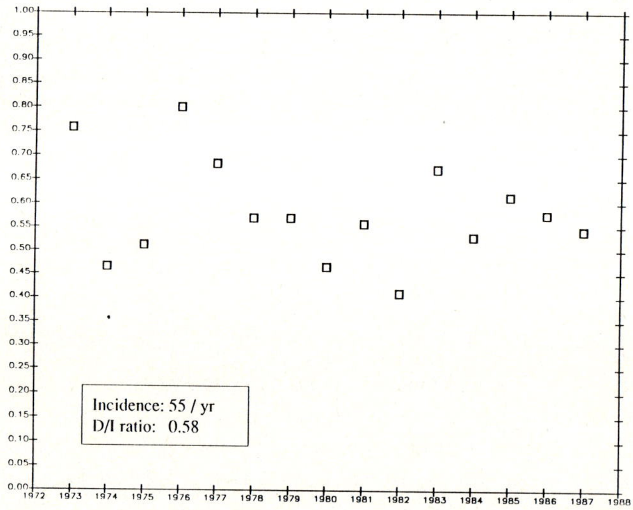

Fig. 5. Cancer of the oropharynx: number of deaths/new cases (death/incidence) in Sweden between 1973 and 1987

mained unchanged during the studied period, but there is an increase in the death rate in patients from France and Germany during the last period. Corresponding analysis from Sweden is shown in Figs 4 and 5. For cancer of the oral cavity, the death rate remained almost unchanged between 1973 and 1987, and the same result was found for cancer of the oropharynx. Thus, therapy has not changed the outcome of disease.

It is very important to analyze risk factors for primary prevention. Boyd (1987) has stressed "that cancer epidemiology seeks ultimately to identify the causes of cancer and thus shares its goals with clinical researchers and laboratory scientists." The following list shows risk factors for cancer of the oral cavity and oropharynx:

1. Tobacco consumption: smoking, snuffing, chewing
2. Marijuana
3. Alcohol
4. Diet
5. Occupational factors
6. Virus infections (human papilloma virus)
7. Genetic instability
8. Aryl hydrocarbon hydroxylase
9. Other

The dominating risk factor is tobacco consumption (through smoking) in combination with alcohol. Smokeless use of tobacco (snuffing and chewing it) is also considered of pathogenic importance, although its role is not yet clear (Hoffmann et al. 1986). Recently, Maier et al. (1991) reviewed occupational risk factors in "blue collar" workers for cancer of the oral cavity and oropharynx, as follows:

1. Man-made mineral vitrous fibers (MMMF)
2. Wool fibers
3. Mustard gas
4. Polymers of vinyl chloride
5. Isopropanyl alcohol
6. Hexavalent chromium
7. Tannin extract
8. Azo dyes

It is very important in such analyses to make adjustments for alcohol and tobacco abuse, because these risk factors may hide other factors. At present, one of the greatest problems is the increase in tobacco consumption in children. In a recent study by the Swedish Health Group (Folkhälsogruppens 1992), it was found that a change in attitude has taken place in 13- to 15-year-olds. During this period, many children are influenced by tobacco company advertisements, and between the ages of 16 and 20, around 40% of children smoke tobacco and/or use it smokelessly (Table 7).

There are different types of analytical epidemiological studies which can be used to identify risk factors in cancer of the oral cavity and oropharynx: interventional, prospective cohort, and retrospective case-control studies. A recently completed Swedish head and neck cancer case-control study was designed to identify risk factors in a defined population (n = 3 million) from

Table 7. Age at first use of tobacco in Sweden (cigarette smoking/smokeless tobacco) (Folkhälsograppens 1992)

Age	Users
11–12 years	Very few
13–15 years	Some
16–20 years	30% users

the area of Stockholm and the Southern Swedish Health Care region. The patients are men aged 40–79 years, were born in Sweden, and have a squamous cell cancer localized to the oral cavity (excluding lip), pharynx (excluding nasopharynx), larynx, or esophagus. Population-based individuals were used as controls, and two nurses worked as professional interviewers.

Very few patients died, and it is considered to be possible to identify risk factors which increase cancer incidence with a factor as low as 2, if 5% of the population is exposed.

References

Boyd NF (1987) The epidemiology of cancer: principles and methods. In: Tannock IF, Hill RP (eds) The basic science of oncology. Pergamon, New York, pp 7–23

Folkhälsogruppens (The Swedish Health Group) (1992) Rapport om tobaksbruk bland unga. Läkartidn 89:1530–1534

Hoffmann D, Harley NK, Fisenne I, Adams JD, Brunnemann KD (1986) Carcinogenic agents in snuff. J Natl Cancer Inst 76:435–437

Jensen OM, Estève J, Moller H, Renard H (1988) Cancer in the European Community and its member states. Eur J Cancer 26:1167–1256

Kurihara M, Aoki K, Hisamicki S (1989) Cancer mortality statistics in the world 1950–1985. The University of Nagoya Press, Nagoya

Maier H, De Vries N, Snow GB (1991) Occupational factors in the etiology of head and neck cancer (a review). Clin Otolaryngol 16:406–412

National Board of Health and Welfare (1988) The Cancer Registry. Cancer Incidence in Sweden

Parkin DM, Lääri E, Muir GS (1988) Estimates of the worldwide frequency of sixteen major cancers in 1980. Int J Cancer 41:184–197

Roland NJ, Caslin AW, Nash J, Stell PM (1992) Value of grading squamous cell carcinoma of the head and neck. Head Neck 14:224–229

Temple NJ, Burkitt DP (1991) The war on cancer—failure of therapy and research: discussion paper. J R Soc Med 84:95–90

Clinical Relevance of Precancerous Lesions of Oral Mucosa

J.J. Pindborg

Department of Oral Pathology and Medicine, School of Dentistry, Faculty of Health Sciences, University of Copenhagen and Dental Department, University Hospital (Rigshospitalet) Copenhagen, Denmark

In 1967, the World Health Organization (WHO) established a WHO Collaborating Centre for Oral Precancerous Lesions in Copenhagen. In 1972, while work was being carried out at this center, a meeting arranged by WHO was held in Geneva with the aim of defining precancerous lesions in different organs of the body. As result of this meeting, the suggestion of distinguishing between precancerous lesions and precancerous conditions was made. A precancerous lesion is a morphologically altered tissue in which cancer is more likely to occur than in its apparently normal counterpart. A precancerous condition, on the other hand, is a generalized state associated with a significantly increased risk of cancer. Examples of precancerous conditions are syphilis, submucous fibrosis, and lichen planus.

This paper will deal only with precancerous lesions, of which there are two: leukoplakia and erythroplakia. In 1978, the WHO Centre published a set of definitions of oral precancer (WHO Collaborating Centre for Oral Precancerous Lesions 1978). A leukoplakia was defined as a white patch or plaque that cannot be characterized clinically or pathologically as any other disease.

This concept broke with the traditional American use of the term leukoplakia as synonymous with epithelial dysplasia. Leukoplakia should only be used as a clinical term. Similarly, the term erythroplakia should be defined as a bright red, velvety plaque which cannot be characterized clinically or pathologically as being due to any other condition.

In 1983, an international seminar was held in Malmö, where the abovementioned definitions were confirmed. Furthermore, it was decided to limit the term leukoplakia. White patches caused by restorative materials, glass blowing, or friction should be termed according to their etiology (Axéll et al. 1984).

Leukoplakia

Clinical Subdivision of Leukoplakia

At the 1983 seminar, it was also suggested that leukoplakias should be clinically classified as homogeneous and nonhomogenous. A homogeneous leukoplakia is a benign, uniformly whitish lesion with a smooth or corrugated surface. Nonhomogeneous leukoplakias (potentially malignant) were divided into: (a) verrucous leukoplakias, (b) nodular leukoplakias, and (c) erythroleukoplakias.

After the Malmö seminar, the author of this paper studied in more detail both the homogeneous and the nonhomogeneous leukoplakias. The result was a revised classification, which is shown in Table 1. A homogeneous leukoplakia may have four different morphologic manifestations often related to etiology. The group of nonhomogeneous lesions has been supplemented with a new entity: the proliferative verrucous leukoplakia, first described by Hansen et al. (1985).

Homogeneous leukoplakias may either be flat, corrugated, wrinkled, or pumice-like in clinical appearance. Homogeneous means that there are no red patches, no nodules, and no verrucous hyperplasias. However, in some patients the homogeneous lesions may have the appearance of cracked mud, but these still belong to the benign type of leukoplakias. Histologic examination shows either hyperortho- or hyperparakeratosis; epithelial dysplasia is rarely seen.

Nonhomogeneous leukoplakias are rarer than the homogeneous types. The nodular leukoplakia and the erythroleukoplakia are the most frequent of the nonhomogeneous types. Originally, the nodular type was termed speckled leukoplakia (Pindborg et al. 1963), but the present author later

Table 1. Clinical classification of oral precancerous lesions

Leukoplakia
Homogeneous
1. Flat
2. Corrugated
3. Pumice-like
4. Wrinkled
Nonhomogeneous
1. Verrucous
2. Proliferative and verrucous
3. Nodular
4. Erythroleutroplakia
Erythroplakia
1. Uniformly red
2. Red with white nodules

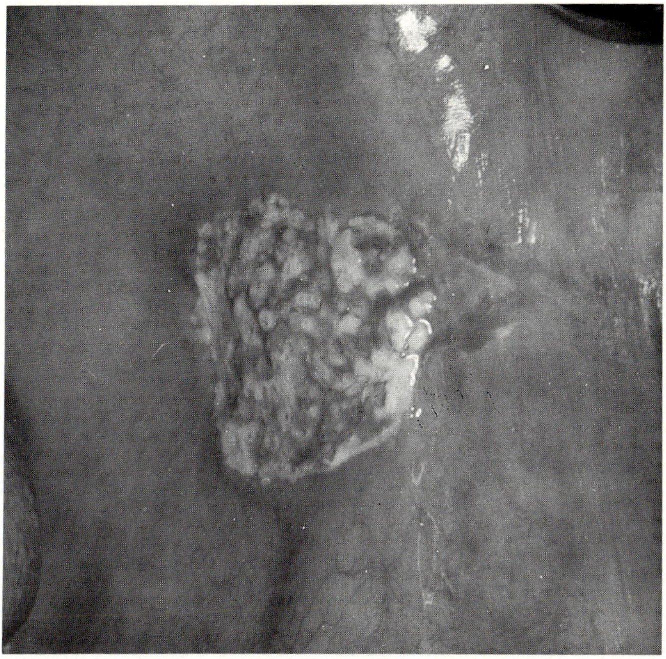

Fig. 1. Typical nodular leukoplakia of left buccal mucosa

realized that the white nodules (Fig. 1) are the most important indicator of impending malignancy and suggested the term nodular leukoplakia (Pindborg 1980). Silverman et al. (1984) emphasized the significance of red (erythroplakic) patches intermingled with white areas (often with nodules) and suggested the very useful term erythroleukoplakia. The nonhomogeneous leukoplakias are almost always the seat of either epithelial dysplasia, carcinoma in situ, or squamous cell carcinoma.

Epidemiologic Consideration

There are a number of epidemiologic studies dealing with the prevalence of leukoplakia (Hogewind and van der Waal 1988). However, most of these studies are only of historical interest, because in most of them no standardized criteria were applied. Two epidemiologic studies have used the classification shown in Table 1. In a study of 20333 adult Swedes, 3.4% had homogeneous leukoplakias and only 0.3% had the nonhomogeneous type (Axéll 1987). A Dutch study of 1000 outpatients in an oral surgery department revealed 0.9% with homogeneous leukoplakias and 0.5% with the nonhomogeneous type (Hogewind 1990; Hogewind and van der Waal 1988).

Clinical Appearance Related to Etiology

At the 1983 seminar, the homogeneous leukoplakias were etiologically divided into those being idiopathic and those associated with tobacco usage. The majority of the idiopathic leukoplakias are of the homogeneous type, but they should always be regularly followed, as some lesions may develop spots of an erythroleukoplakia.

With regard to tobacco, leukoplakias may be caused by either smoking or smokeless tobacco. Tobacco has a specific effect upon the oral epithelium. Clinically, the tobacco-induced leukoplakias may present with a pumice-like appearance and a morphology similar to fingerprints (Fig. 2). Histologically, the "fingerprints" have a specific keratinization, the so-called chevron type of keratinization (Pindborg et al. 1980). In 1973, the pumice pattern was described under the name of "cigarette smoker's lip lesion" (Berry and Landwerlen 1973).

The same changes may be observed in snuff-induced lesions, especially in those located on the lower labial mucosa. However, most snuff-induced lesions are characterized by a wrinkling of the mucosa. The presence of wrinkling (from mild to heavy) of the mucosa has been used to grade snuff-

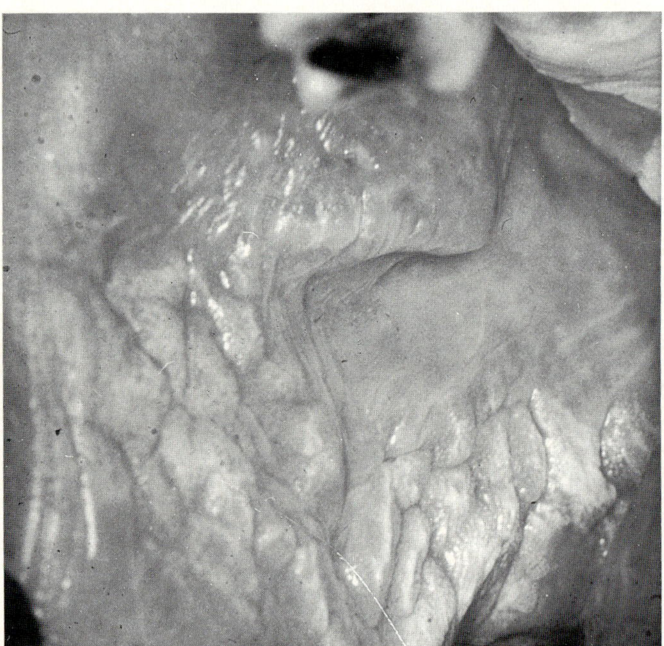

Fig. 2. Pumice-like leukoplakia. Note finger-print-like changes of mucosa in a heavy smoker

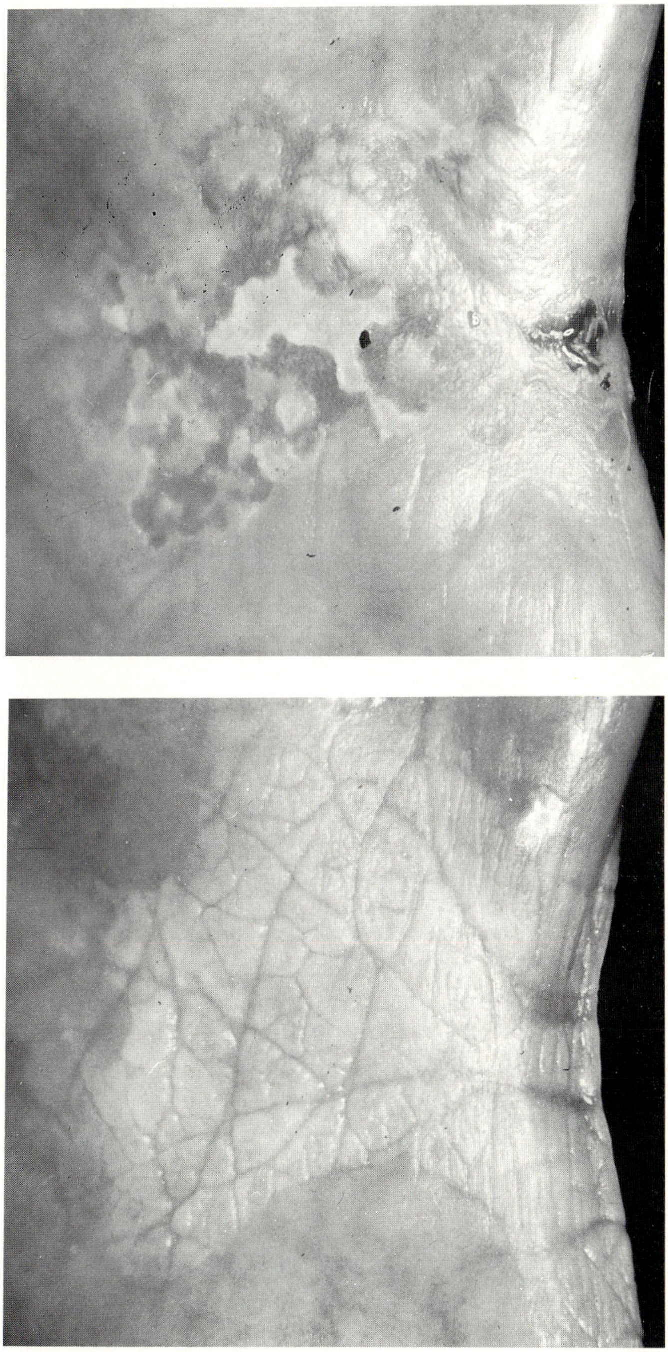

A

B

Fig. 3. **A** Erythroleukoplakia in left commissure of heavy smoker. **B** Six weeks later after application (four times a day) of nystatin vaginals

induced lesions. A Swedish study (Axéll et al. 1976) used a four-degree scale, which has been modified by investigators in USA to comprise only three stages (Greer and Poulson 1983).

In recent years, several studies have emphasized the presence of *Candida albicans* in leukoplakias. Thus, Cawson and Lehner (1968) have suggested the term candidal leukoplakia. *Candida*-infected leukoplakias are often the seat of ulcerations.

In the experience of the author, most, if not all, nonhomogeneous leukoplakias are the seat of a *Candida* infection. It has been demonstrated that a nodular leukoplakia can be transformed into a homogeneous leukoplakia (Holmstrup and Bessermann 1983). Figure 3 illustrates that an erythroleukoplakia can also be transformed into a homogeneous leukoplakia using antifungals.

Clinical Appearance as a Predictor

The distinction between homogeneous and nonhomogeneous leukoplakia is based on two features: (1) demonstration of a higher prevalence of epithelial dysplasia in nonhomogeneous leukoplakia compared with homogeneous lesions and (2) the higher rate of malignant transformation from nonhomogeneous leukoplakias. The latter has been demontrated in studies in Germany (Maerker and Burkhardt 1978; Tischendorf and Giehler 1990), Hungary (Bánóczy 1977), and the USA (Silverman et al. 1984). The results of a follow-up study in India are shown in Table 2. It is obvious that the nodular leukoplakia is a very dangerous lesion with a high risk of malignant transformation.

The pumice-like leukoplakia caused by tobacco usage is a benign lesion, apparently with no malignant potential (Pindborg et al. 1980). When tobacco usage is stopped, it is very often reversible. Only when it becomes infected with *Candida* does it change its potential. This change is due to the fact that *Candida albicans*, when present in oral leukoplakias, contributes to

Table 2. Malignant potential of oral precancer (after Gupta et al. 1989)

Precursor lesion/condition	Total (*n*)	Average follow up period (years)	Oral cancers (*n*)	Relative risk
Nodular leukoplakia	13	2.8	6	3243
Submucous fibrosis	25	6.0	3	8397
Red areas, ulcers	26	2.6	1	303
Ulcerated leukoplakia	105	4.4	1	44
Homogeneous leukoplakia	489	4.8	3	26
Lichen planus	344	3.7	1	16
None of the above	10145	7.8	4	1

the production of carcinogenic nitrosamines (Krogh et al. 1987). These findings open up new avenues in our understanding of the malignant potential of leukoplakias.

Erythroplakia

The other oral precancerous lesion, the erythroplakia, is much rarer than leukoplakia. However, in contrast to leukoplakia, it is always associated with epithelial dysplasia, carcinoma in situ, or carcinoma (Shafer and Waldron 1975). The same investigators found that carcinomas were observed 17 times more frequently in erythroplakia than in leukoplakia lesions.

References

Axéll T (1987) Occurrence of leukoplakia and some other oral white lesions among 20333 adult Swedish people. Community Dent Oral Epidemiol 15:46–51

Axéll T, Mörnstad H, Sundström B (1976) The relation of the clinical picture to the histopathology of snuff dipper's lesions in a Swedish population. J Oral Pathol 5:229–236

Axéll T, Holmstrup P, Kramer IRH, Pindborg JJ, Shear M (1984) International seminar on oral leukoplakia and associated lesions to tobacco habits. Community Dent Oral Epidemial 12:145–154

Bánóczy J (1977) Follow-up studies in oral leukoplakia. J Max Fac Surg 5:69–75

Berry HH, Landwerlen JR (1973) Cigarette smoker's lip lesion in psychiatric patients. J Am Dent Assoc 86:657–662

Cawson RA, Lehner T (1968) Chronic hyperplastic candidiasis–candidal leukoplakia. Br J Dermatol 80:9–16

Greer RO, Poulson TC (1983) Oral tissue alterations associated with the use of smokeless tobacco by teenagers. Oral Surg Oral Med Oral Pathol 56:275–284

Gupta PC, Bhonsle RB, Murti PR, Daftary DK, Mehta FS, Pindborg JJ (1989) An epidemiologic assessment of cancer risk in oral precancerous lesions in India with special reference to nodular leukoplakia, Cancer 63:2247–2252

Hansen LS, Olson JA, Silverman S JR (1985) Proliferative verrucous leukoplakia. Oral Surg Oral Med Pathol 60:285–298

Hogewind WFC (1990) Oral leukoplakia in a Dutch population: a clinical study. Thesis, University of Amsterdam

Hogewind WFC, van der Waal I (1988) Prevalence study of oral leukoplakia in a selected population of 1000 patients from the Netherlands. Community Dent Oral Epidemiol 16:302–305

Holmstrup P, Bessermann M (1983) Clinical, therapeutic, and pathogenic aspects of chronic oral multifocal candidiasis. Oral Surg Oral Med Oral Pathol 56:388–396

Krogh D, Hald B, Holmstrup P (1987) Possible mycological etiology of oral mucosal cancer: catalytic potential of infecting *Candida albicans* and other yeasts in production of N-nitrosobenzylmethylamine. Carcinogenesis 8:1543–1548

Maerker R, Burkhardt A (1978) Klinik der oralen Leukoplakien und Präkanzerosen. Retrospektive Studie on 200 Patienten. Dtsch Z Mund Kiefer Gesichtschir 2: 206–220

Pindborg JJ (1980) Oral cancer and precancer. Wright, Bristol

Pindborg JJ, Renstrup G, Poulsen HE, Silverman S Jr. (1963) Studies in oral leukoplakias: V. Clinical and histologic signs of malignancy. Acta Odontol Scand 21:407–414

Pindborg JJ, Reibel J, Roed-Petersen B, Mehta FS (1980) Tobacco-induced changes in oral leukoplakic epithelium. Cancer 45:2333–2336

Shafer WG, Waldron CA (1975) Erythroplakias of the oral cavity. Cancer 36: 1021–1028

Silverman S Jr, Goisky M, Lozada F (1984) Oral leukoplakia and malignant transformation. A follow-up study of 257 patients. Cancer 53:563–568

Tischendorf L, Giehler U (1990) Studien zur Dignität der Leukoplakien von Mundschleimhaut und Lippen. Dtsch Z Mund Kiefer Gesichtschir 14:301–305

WHO Collaborating Centre for Oral Precancerous Lesions (1978) An aid to studies on oral precancer. Oral Surg Oral Med Oral Pathol 46:518–539

Extended Surgery for Advanced Maxillary Sinus Carcinoma

P.J. Donald

Department of Otolaryngology – Head and Neck Surgery, University of California, Davis, USA

Maxillary sinus carcinoma is a relatively uncommon head and neck tumor. It makes up 3% of head and neck malignancies. The commonest histology is squamous cell carcinoma, although adenoid cystic carcinoma, acinic cell tumor, and adenocarcinoma are not uncommon. These are primarily epithelial neoplasms arising in the mucosal lining of the sinus. Primary tumors of bone such as osteogenic sarcoma, ameloblastoma, and chondrosarcoma arise in the skeletal elements of the sinus. Consideration must also be given to those malignancies that arise from adjacent tissue and invade the maxilla and the maxillary sinus by direct extension. Examples of these are aggressive and neurotropic skin tumors such as basal cell carcinoma, squamous cell carcinoma, and malignant melanoma, which may invade the maxilla by extending along the vascular and neural foramina of the orbit and maxillary face. Direct extension of oral cavity tumors, such as carcinoma of the alveolar ridge, and nasal cavity tumors, such as esthesioneuroblastoma, and inferior extension of ethmoidal malignancies further exemplify spread from contiguous sites.

The maxillary sinus is like a six-sided box, with each side facing a distinctly different anatomical area, which, when invaded, will show characteristic, identifiable symtoms (Fig. 1). Expansion of the floor produces dental protrusion, a mass or ulcer in the alveolus, or an ill-fitting denture. Erosion of tumor through the anterior wall produces fullness, swelling, pain, skin ulceration, and infraorbital nerve hypesthesia (an ominous sign). Medial wall protrusion results in epistaxis, purulent nasal drainage, obstruction to breathing, and even bulging of the nasal framework. Superior extension invokes orbital symptoms ranging from pressure, pain, and epiphora to diplopia, blindness, and proptosis.

Lateral and posterior extension produce symptoms of more subtlety such as numbness over the maxillary branch of the trigeminal nerve or trismus. A presenting symptom may even be serous otitis media from spread through

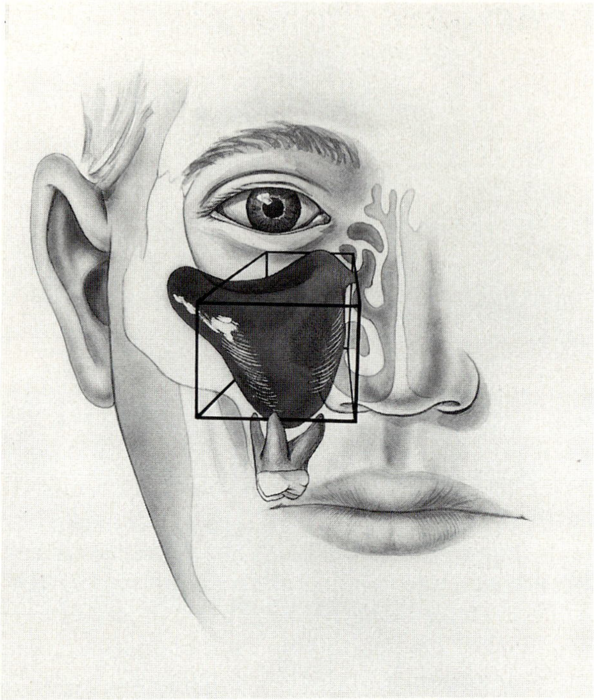

Fig. 1. Maxillary sinus sits like a six-sided box. Spread from any side will produce uniquely characteristic symptoms. (From Thawley and Panje 1987)

the posterior wall to the pterygomaxillary space and then on to the nasopharynx.

Occasionally, carcinomas in the maxillary sinus suprastructure may invade more superiorly than inferiorly and thereby grow through the ethmoids bone and thus into the anterior cranial fossa. Similarly, ethmoidal and nasal cavity tumors may descend into the superior maxilla. Ethmoid extensions may proceed laterally into the orbit and, if near the apex, cross into the middle cranial fossa.

The primary consideration in this paper is the management of extensive tumors. Traditionally, Ohngren's line divided the maxillary sinus into two roughly triangular spaces. The anteroinferior space tumors have been generally thought of having a reasonably acceptable prognosis with a 5-year survival rate of around 60%. Conversely, those of the so-called suprastructure were thought to have such a poor prognosis that some authorities advised against aggressive surgery.

The advent of skull base surgery has markedly changed the outlook for those unfortunate victims of advanced sinus malignancy. Traditional relative contraindications to maxillectomy such as symptoms of blindness, trismus, and numbness of the trigeminal branches are no longer considered as such. Findings of posterior wall and pterygoid plate invasion, pterygoid muscle involvement, erosion of the optic canal, invasion of the sphenoid bone or sphenoid sinus, transgression of the anterior or middle cranial fossa, extension into the cavernous sinus, or involvement of the nasopharynx and clivus once almost universally accepted as absolute contra-indications to surgery are now considered by many skull base surgeons as surmountable problems. Dural and even cerebral invasion are not thought of by some as impediments to complete surgical extirpation of disease in selected patients.

The Skull Base Surgical Team

Skull base surgery is the combined cooperative effort of the head and neck surgeon and the neurological surgeon. The successful execution of these complex, time-consuming, and sometimes hazardous procedures requires absolute synchrony between these two principals. If neither surgeon is well versed in reconstructive techniques such as calvarial bone grafting, myocutaneous or free flap reconstruction, then the expertise of a plastic surgeon is sought.

A preoperative meeting to discuss the management of each individual case facilitates mutual understanding of each surgeon's role in the preoperative assessment, the use of perioperative adjuncts such as lumbar subarachnoid drainage or brain protection with barbiturate coma, the placement of incisions, the timing and sequencing of each phase of the operative procedure, preparations for possible unforeseen problems, and the type of reconstruction. A review of computerized axial tomography (CAT) scans, magnetic resonance imaging (MRI), angiograms, carotid balloon test occlusion (when relevant), and a discussion of the histology are an integral part of the assessment.

Procedures

The simplest procedure involves resection of tumors of the suprastructure of the maxilla with ethmoid, and often orbital and intracranial, extension.

A lateral rhinotomy is done and the anterior face of the maxillary sinus exposed. The periorbita is dissected laterally if uninvolved with the tumor. If limited periorbital invasion is found and in a relatively unaggressive tumor, it is probably safe in some cases to resect the periorbita and some adjacent periorbital fat, thereby preserving the globe. In cases of more extensive involvement, orbital exenteration is carried out. However, an important caveat must supervene: If doubt exists, resect the eye. A heroic attempt to save the eye, but risk the patient's life, is foolhardy. A coiplete ethmoidectomy and a Denker operation on the maxillary sinus are performed for exposure.

During this part of the procedure in bulky tumors, a large portion of the tumor may have to be excised piecemeal in order to provide adequate visualization. Some objections to piecemeal resection have been raised because of the traditional notion that such excision will seed tumor cells throughout the operative site. In the author's 17-year experience of such excisions, this has not been found to be the case. Local recurrence rates following piecemeal excision are little different from those reported for en bloc resection. A further objection to this technique is the problem of the awareness of margins. A serious obligation is imposed upon the surgeon using this technique to be constantly vigilant as to the margin of resection. The overwhelming advantages of the removal of tumor obtundation of vital structures and deep tumor extension allowing a narrower approach and conservation of normal uninvolved tissue far outweigh the tedium of constantly being aware of resection margins. As already mentioned, the theoretical objection to tumor seeding is ill-founded.

Once the medial maxilla and ethmoid bone have been exenterated, the eye transected at the apex (when indicated), and visual obscuring by tumor is cleared, then an assessment of the remaining structures involved can be done. Tumor penetration of the anterior fossa floor is left undisturbed. Sphenoid extension is assessed and the anterior wall of the sinus removed. Clival involvement, penetration of the lateral sphenoid sinus wall into cavernous sinus, and involvement of the optic nerve in the optic canal and the maxillary branch of the trigeminal nerve at the foramen rotundum are assessed. Rarely in cases of malignancy is there posterior maxillary sinus wall penetration and pterygoid muscle involvement that does not mandate total maxillectomy.

An inferiorly placed frontal craniotomy is done, the height of which is usually predicated according to anterior fossa tumor extent, as determined from below, together with the assessment of the preoperative scans. In certain cases of limited anterior extent, an osteoplastic flap of the anterior frontal sinus wall with removal of the posterior wall may be performed. The sinus is cranialized at the completion of the case.

An intradural or extradural exposure is done, depending on the preference of the neurosurgeon, but often based on presence and degree of intradural invasion. Intracerebral invasion is fortunately rare and obviously requires intradural exposure.

Intracranial control is carried out by dissection, even as far posteriorly as the lesser sphenoid wing and the planum sphenoidale. The olfactory bulbs are often sacrificed when tumor involves the nasal vault; once the dural involvement by tumor is circumscribed and adjacent dural margins are histologically negative on frozen section, the remaining brain and dura are protected by the neurosurgeon as the head and neck surgeon outlines the tumor penetration of the anterior fossa floor from below. Being vigilant to maintain the integrity of tumor-free margins, the head and neck surgeon uses a long 2- or 3-mm osteotome and light mallet taps to entirely encompass the disease as it encroaches upon or penetrates the floor. Once loosened, the specimen is delivered from above down through the facial wound. Margins are checked by multiple frozen sections at the resection edge.

Certain key areas are targeted for frozen section analysis. The optic nerve as it emerges from its canal is sectioned. A margin may not be obtained until the chiasm is reached intracranially. The stump of the maxillary branch of the trigeminal nerve is examined. If positive as it emerges from the foramen rotundum, the bone of the foraminal edge is drilled away with a cutting bur until middle fossa dura is encountered and a sample of nerve taken flush with dura that is negative. A positive margin mandates resection into the middle cranial fossa. The cranial nerves as they emerge from the superior orbital fissure are similarly biopsied. Further tumor involvement in the sphenoidal contribution to the skull base usually only occurs under circumstances when the entire maxilla requires removal. The closure will be discussed at the completion of the discussion on total maxillectomy.

When the infrastructure is invaded or the tumor begins at this site and progresses superiorly, a total maxillectomy is required. A Weber-Fergusson incision is used, the lip split and the facial skin dissected laterally. Soft tissue, including skin invasion, is included with a wide margin of surrounding healthy tissue. This stands in stark contrast to the mere 1- to 2-mm margins required in cranial nerves or 2- to 4-mm margins in dura. The maxilla, usually with the eye, is resected in the standard fashion, usually initially leaving behind a small triangular area that is the remnant of the posterior maxillary sinus wall. This wall and the adjacent pterygoid plates are removed with the cutting bur, and the soft tissue with resection forceps. The internal maxillary artery will require control with a clip, ligature, or bipolar cautery.

Pterygoid muscle involvement mandates resection to the insertion of the muscles on the mandible. For extra insurance, the periosteum at the site of insertion is included. Resecting less than this is an invitation to local recurrence.

Invasion of the peritubal muscles and the eustachian tube can be resected to a limited extent from this approach. More extensive involvement requires exposure through the middle fossa combined with infratemporal fossa approach because of safety in controlling the internal carotid artery and the inability to get beyond the impediments posed by the mandible and the masticatory muscles. Extension into nasopharyngeal vault mucosa and clivus can be controlled by sharp dissection and the cutting bur.

The undersurface of the body of the sphenoid bone may be partially eroded by tumor and was formerly considered to be a criterion of inoperability. Of all the prior criteria of surgical hopelessness, this is the most puzzling. The bone is very thick, widely exposed with the maxilla and orbital contents removed, and it is relatively simple to distinguish between involved and uninvolved bone when removing it with a bur. The bone is removed, keeping in mind the position of the foramen ovale and the relative proximity of the internal carotid artery. Limited access to the cavernous sinus is afforded, but it can usually be adequately controlled to resect tumors that have invaded it.

Closure begins after all loose and stray bits of bone are removed, sharp protruding edges are drilled away, hemostasis has been secured, and all frozen sections have been sent to pathology, insuring a complete resection. Dural dehiscences are patched with fasciae or lyophilized dura. A watertight seal is striven for. An inferiorly pedicled pericranial flap is tucked over the lower cut edge of the craniotomy and stretches over the defect in the anterior fossa floor. There is no necessity for bony reconstruction of the anterior fossa floor. A split thickness skin graft lines the cavity and is kept in place with gauze packing. A dental prosthesis is placed in cases of radical maxillectomy. Skin closure is done in the usual fashion with fine nylon sutures. The lumbar drain is usually out in 72 h. Packing and sutures are removed under general anesthesia at the end of the first postoperative week. The tracheostomy is usually corked the day after packing removal and removed the following day.

Extended Anterior Resection

In unusually extensive lesions, some that even originate in the pharyngeal mucosa, have both maxillary and mandibular involvement. In addition, facial skin and even the parotid gland may be involved. With both the condyle and the ramus of the mandible and the maxilla removed, a complete exposure of the undersurface of the middle fossa floor is possible. With foramen ovale and foramen spinosum exposed and the cartilaginous eustachian tube identified medially, the anterior and undersurface of the temporal bone as well its medial articulation with the sphenoid can be removed with the cutting bur.

Indeed the internal carotid artery can be exposed all the way from the neck through the petrosa, cavernous sinus and into the circle of Willis (Fig. 2). The cavernous sinus can be safely resected, as well as the anterior pole of the temporal lobe and dura (Fig. 3). Such resections can proceed down the clivus almost to the foramen magnum.

During the reconstructive phase, separation of the intracranial contents from the upper aerodigestive tract usually requires the use of a musculocutaneous free flap. The latissimus dorsomusculo-cutaneous free flap provides sufficient bulk as well as an excellent vascular pedicle. The flap acts to improve appearance somewhat, filling in the huge defect left by the resection, and neatly separates the intracranial cavity from the nasopharynx and oral cavity. The major problem is the possible effacement of early detection

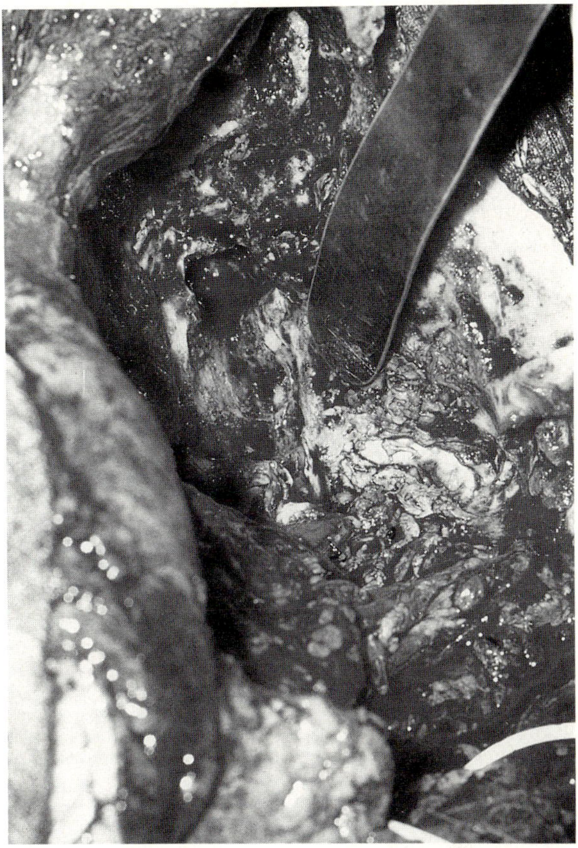

Fig. 2. Close-up view of extensive anterior transfacial subcranial approach. Retractor is against temporal lobe dura. Medially is the internal carotid artery whose petrosal course can be seen inferior to the retractor. Medial to the cavernous carotid artery is the exenterated sphenoidal sinus

if recurrent tumor should emerge. Unfortunately, the CAT scan and MRI are often unable to distinguish early recurrence because of the changes wrought by postoperative fibrosis and the effects of radiation.

The survival rates after surgery of paranasal malignancies that transgress the skull base are included in the overall survival rate for the tumors that involve the anterior fossa floor. They do, however, make up the major contribution to this group. Only a few tumors extend as far back as the middle fossa. In 1991, the author undertook a national survey in the USA of all skull base centers performing this surgery for malignant disease. Among the institutions reporting, there were 153 cases of cancer invading the anterior fossa and 437 cases involving the middle fossa. The 2-year and better

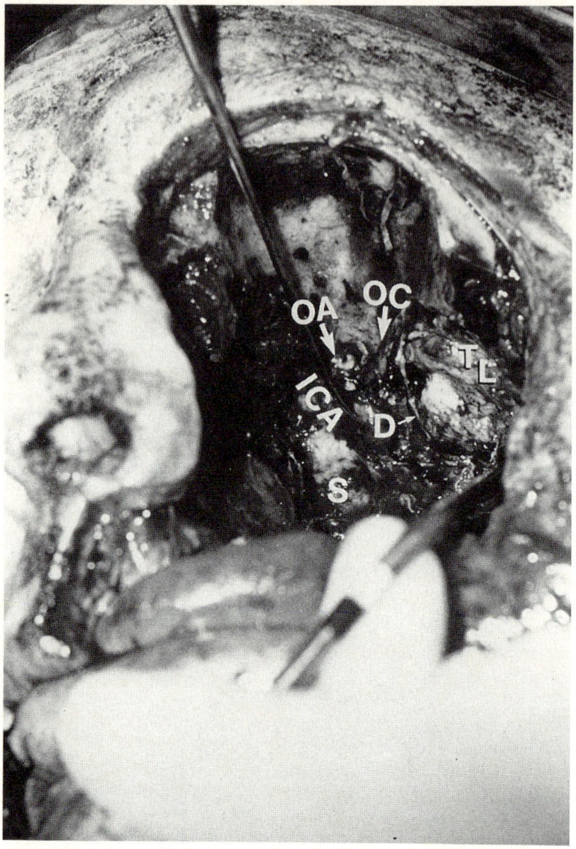

Fig. 3. Anterior transfacial subcranial approach used to resect a large, highly invasive squamous cell carcinoma of the maxillary and ethmoid sinuses. *OA*, ophthalmic artery; *OC*, optic canal with optic nerve; *TL*, temporal lobe; *D*, temporal lobe dura; *S*, sphenoid sinus; *ICA*, internal carotid artery

disease-free survival rate was 60% for the anterior fossa and 47% for the middle fossa. Clearly the survival figures of these patients is certainly worth the effort in removing their otherwose deadly tumor.

Reference

Thawley SE, Panje WR (eds) (1987) Comprehensive management of head and neck tumors. Saunders, Philadelphia

Resection of Tumors in Tongue, Floor of the Mouth, and Mandible: Possibilities of Primary Reconstruction

J.-E. Hausamen and F.W. Neukam

Klinik und Poliklinik für Mund-, Kiefer- und Gesichtschirurgie, Medizinische Hochschule Hannover, Konstanty-Gutschow-Str. 8, 30625 Hannover, Germany

Introduction

In the surgical treatment of maxillofacial tumors, the same basic requirements have to be fulfilled as in the surgical treatment of tumors located in other regions of the body. This means early and complete removal of the tumor by radical tumor resection, in the case of malignant tumors even removal of the regional lymphatic drainage area.

The damage caused by tumor resection may be restricted to a small local area, but it can also be very extensive, involving soft tissue and facial bones, and can also produce functional disturbances by destroying the continuity of sensory and motor nerves. In one respect, resection of maxillofacial tumors decisively differs from tumor surgery in other regions of the body: it produces changes in the face which the patient himself and his relatives often consider to be deforming.

An intact face is of utmost importance for the self-esteem and self-confidence of a patient and plays a most significant role in human relations. Consequently, the maxillofacial surgeon must not simply deal with the local problems of a tumor and strive for permanent healing by radical resection. At the same time he should also aim at restoring form and function and consider any therapeutic measure under the aspect of facial esthetics.

Unfortunately, we have not succeeded in considerably increasing the survival rates of patients following resection of malignant tumors over the last 20 years, although tremendous efforts have been made to increase surgical radicality and employ various forms of chemotherapy or radiotherapy. However, we have made considerable progress in reconstructive measures by developing new techniques which enable extensive, radical tumor resection without permanent deformation of the patient.

Adequate repair of defects produced by tumor resection in the face is possible only if the soft tissue involved, the supporting bony structures and also the function are fully restored. Thanks to the progress made in maxillofacial surgery, we are now in the position to repair all these structures, i.e., facial soft tissue, facial skeleton, and sensory and motor nerves. Thus, even after radical tumor resection, patients are able to live a normal life in our society. A considerable step forward in this respect was the introduction of microsurgery several years ago. Microsurgical techniques have significantly improved the results in the restoration of nerves, and microvascular surgery enables utilization of an unlimited amount of well-vascularized soft tissue and bone grafts (Riediger et al. 1986; Neukam et al. 1987, 1989, 1990; Hausamen and Neukam 1992).

Treatment of Carcinomas of the Oral Cavity

Carcinomas of the oral cavity, especially carcinomas of the floor of the mouth and tongue, often require extensive resection of oral mucosa. The replacement of oral mucosa has presented one major problem: because of the limited supply of mucosa from the oral cavity itself, only minor defects could be repaired by end-to-end reconstruction or by local transposition flaps from the palate, the cheek, or the tongue.

Small, noninvasive T1 tumors of the tongue with a maximum diameter of 2 cm can be resected in all three dimensions with an extented surgical margin of 1.5–2 cm, and the resulting soft tissue defect can be closed by primary adaptation. Such localized resections should be performed in tumors involving the lateral border, the dorsum, and the tip of the tongue.

Localized T1 and T2 tumors which are situated more sublingually or with extension to the floor of the mouth, can also be resected in all three dimensions with partial resection of the floor of the mouth, eventually with marginal resection of the mandible. Even in such cases, a local reconstruction of the defect by primary adaptation of the surgical margins of the tongue with the mandibular gingiva or a mucoperiosteal flap from the vestibulum can be recommended.

In T3 and T4-tumors extending to the floor of the mouth, a hemiglossectomy and, in the case of mandibular involvement, a partial or hemimandibulectomy is quite often necessary. Depending on the extension of the tumor, parts of the soft palate or the lateral pharyngeal wall have to be resected. In former times, intraoral reconstruction of the defect was performed by adaptation of the palatal mucosa and the lateral pharyngeal wall with the base of the tongue and by stepwise closure of the remaining tongue with intraoral soft tissue and buccal mucosa. Such a soft tissue reconstruction resulted in postoperative dislocation of the tongue and enormous functional disturbances.

Accordingly, reconstructive techniques were sought that enable the surgeon to perform primary reconstruction of the tissue defect of the tongue and floor of the mouth even in large tumor defects. In former years, the grafting of skin in the form of pedicle flaps from the forehead, breast, or shoulder was the preferred method to cover such extensive defects. Shrinkage and fibrosis of the grafted skin could not be influenced and often led to functional disturbances with restricted mouth opening. Furthermore, the skin is unable to functionally adjust to the oral environment, resulting in further unfavorable consequences of skin grafts such as the continuous secretion of sebaceous glands, desquamation of keratinizing epithelium, and unrestricted growth of hairs.

A decisive step forward was made by microvascular surgery, in particular the introduction of free jejunal grafts, as described by Reuther and Steinau in 1980. Such grafts were the first to meet the requirement of a mucosal replacement of high functional quality, and their availability was practically unlimited. Jejunum and its mesentery harvested at the level of the fourth arcade are used to replace oral mucosa.

After systematization of this surgical method, we have used jejunal grafts quite frequently and have repaired all larger soft tissue defects in the cheek, the soft palate, the tongue, and the oral floor.

Jejunal grafts without reconstruction of maxillary bone or external skin are only performed in isolated tumors of the soft palate, the tongue, or the cheek. In such cases, however, access to the tumor site is often only possible by temporarily splitting the mandible.

The jejunal graft is harvested by a general surgeon. Normally, the graft has the length of a vascular arcade. The jejunum is opened electrosurgically opposite the mesentery. Length and shape of the jejunal graft are fashioned extracorporally. If a smaller graft is required than that harvested, the mesenteric vessels are ligated, but the mesentery is used for padding the soft tissue. Subsequently, the excessive jejunal tissue is cut off. Placement of the graft into the recipient site always has to take account of the individual requirements, and the jejunal graft can made to fit the defect and folded to form a body of tongue.

For arterial anastomosis, all branches of the external carotid artery may be used, as their diameters largely correspond to the diameter of the mesenteric artery. For venous anastomosis, too, suitable vessels are available, provided no neck dissection has been done. In the case of a neck dissection, we use the superior thyroid vein for anastomosis so that drainage is ensured via the thyroid gland. The usual techniques of microvascular anastomosis are used.

In composite or perforating defects we use free jejunal grafts in combination with bone and – if necessary – skin transplants. For the latter we use the standardized techniques of reconstruction (Fig. 1).

Functional Results

We have now used free jejunal grafts to reconstruct extensive mucosal defects of the tongue and floor of the mouth in more than 120 patients. We

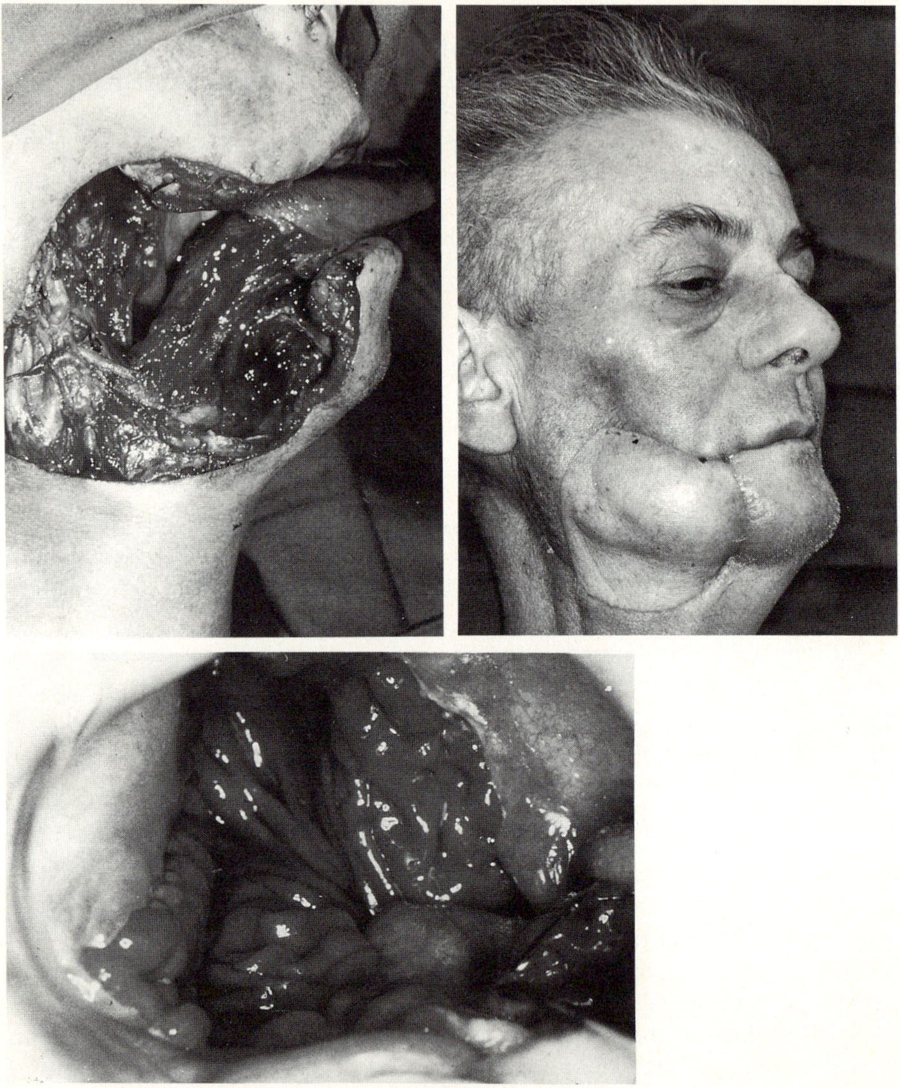

a c b

Fig. 1a–c. Reconstruction of a perforating defect of the cheek. **a** A 55-year-old male with carcinoma of mandible and cheek that had perforated into the extraoral soft tissue, causing a large perforation. **b** Reconstruction of tongue and floor of the mouth by a jejunal graft. The entire left floor of the mouth, the mandibular and buccal lining, and a large area of the soft palate have been repaired by jejunal mucosa; the intestinal folds have become flat and straight and the tongue remained mobile. **c** The buccal skin was repaired by an acromiopectoral flap, and the mandible using alloplastic material

have evaluated the functional results of this special reconstructive technique of tongue and floor of mouth defects for the German Cancer Congress this year in Berlin. In cooperation with the Department of Phoniatrics, the mobility of the tongue and floor of the mouth was investigated using sonography, and speech ability was objectified using tape recordings of standardized single words.

This study resulted in interesting findings which led us to modify our indication for free jejunal grafts.

We have found the best speech results in cases of sagittal resection of lateral parts of the tongue and floor of the mouth reaching the dimension of a hemiglossectomy. In these cases, the defect reconstruction from a close vicinity and reconstruction with a jejunal graft resulted in ideal speech results. With the mobility of the jejunal graft and the function of the remaining tongue, speech results could be achieved that were quite comparable to those of normal controls. However, a transplant volume of more than half of the tongue clearly worsened the speech results. Apparently, the remaining tongue musculature is not able to adequately move the larger transplant volume. An ideal indication for jejunal grafts also exists for tumors of the lateral base of the tongue extending to the soft palate or the lateral pharyngeal wall. For this site, the jejunal graft is superior to all other reconstructive techniques, because it can be excellently adapted to the specific anatomical structures of the soft palate and the lateral pharyngeal wall and, therefore, allows undisturbed motion of the tongue.

However, following transversal resection of the anterior third of the tongue and the anterior floor of the mouth with jejunal reconstruction, the functional speech results were clearly worse than after sagittal resections of the lateral parts of the tongue. Even in cases of subtotal transverse glossectomies followed by free jejunal graft reconstruction, the functional speech results were not satisfying. Due to missing volume, the jejunal graft is apparently unable to provide a sufficient closure towards the palate.

Therefore, we have started to use voluminous, microvascular, cutaneous or myocutaneous transplants for extensive resections of large parts of the tongue, especially located anteriorly, thus allowing passive closure between transplant and palate. Particulary in slim patients, the free rectus abdominis flap or the radial forearm flap proved to be optimal, being easier to fit the palatal concavity by molding in a cylindrical fashion.

Reconstruction of the Mandible

Most problems connected with bone grafting have now been solved, since the introduction of microvascular bone grafting has considerably increased the indications for bone grafting and has made available grafting material of high biological quality. The goal aimed at by reconstruction of the facial bones is not simply the anatomic restoration of the bony structures, but also restoration of masticatory function. Dental replacement in the form of dental implants has opened up a wide field of possibilities which were still inconceivable only a few years ago before the problems of long-term anchorage of the implant in free and microvascular bone grafts was solved.

It is possible to replace bone by free corticocancellous bone grafts, cancellous bone chips, or microvascular bone transplants. Free autogenous bone is now unanimously considered the best material to replace bone (Reichenbach et al. 1957; Rehrmann 1955, 1978).

The quality of the recipient area is of decisive importance for selecting the bone to be grafted, since the survival of a free bone graft depends on the supply of the grafted bone, first by diffusion and subsequently by quick vascularization. The latter processes are influenced by the quality of the recipient site, i.e., intact periosteum and well-vascularized muscular tissue are very favorable in this respect (Lexer 1908). Chronically infected tissue or tissue previously submitted to irradiation are not favorable. Free bone grafting to such unfavorable recipient sites is only possible under certain conditions, since supply of the graft by diffusion and subsequent quick vascularization is not guaranteed. For these unfavorable recipient sites we now have the alternative of microvascular reanastomosed bone grafts, which guarantees vitality of the entire graft, provided that sufficient vascular anastomoses are possible (Taylor et al. 1975, 1979; Salibian et al. 1985; Riediger 1988).

In contrast to free bone grafts, the healing of microvascular reanastomosed bone grafts is not influenced by the quality of the recipient site and is comparable to normal fracture healing. If microsurgically revascularized bone is grafted, a solid bony connection between recipient bone and graft may be assumed to exist 4 weeks postoperatively, so that loading is possible after 4–6 weeks at the latest.

In partial resection of the mandible, a distinction is made between defects in the lateral region of the mandible and defects in the clin portion. Loss of the lateral mandibular body with subsequent bagging out of the lower buccal region is an esthetic impairment that can generally be tolerated, with mandibular function being largely maintained by the contralateral intact part of the mandible. Resection of the central part, i.e., of the chin, however, may result in a threat to life directly after resection if the loss of structures supporting the musculature of the oral floor and tongue makes the body of the tongue fall back and thus produces peripheral breathing disturbances. In order to maintain vital functions, the immediate reconstruction of the chin region is therefore absolutely necessary, while restoration of the lateral mandibular body is not particularly urgent and may be done without in exceptional cases.

Today, in the case of benign tumors of the mandible, we replace bone immediately, preferably by free bone grafts from the iliac crest. The loss of large parts of the mandibular body is easily compensated by such grafts, since contouring and cutting the free iliac bone allows individual reconstruction of the mandible in its original form. Particular shaping and placing of the end of the free graft into the fossa even allows replacement of the mandibular condyle, so that early function of the temporomandibular joint is guaranteed, including more or less normal mouth opening. In small defects, miniplates are used to fix the grafts to the jaw stumps. These miniplates provide sufficient stability of the graft, clearly minimize traumatization of the transplant, and allow early functional loading of the bone graft.

In malignant tumors, we do not use primary bone grafting. Instead, we replace the mandible by plates bridging the defect. The plates keep the jaw stumps in position and can be lined or padded with Palacos or Silastic for better contouring. As an alternative to temporary alloplastic replacement of the mandible, free autogenous rib grafts may be used. Because of the often poor condition of the recipient site, insufficient bony remodeling is likely to occur, often resulting in fractures of the rib grafts. Therefore, osteomyocutaneous pedicle flaps using the pectoralis major muscle are also recommended for primary replacement of the mandible, their advantage being the guaranteed blood supply (Cuono and Ariyan 1988). These pedicled rib grafts are not very easily resorbed, so they can be used even in regions exposed to mechanical load and recipient sites of poor general condition.

Only after the patient has been free of recurrence for 1–2 years is the alloplastic replacement or temporary rib graft replaced by a final, high-quality bone graft from the iliac crest. The surgical techniques applied in secondary mandibular replacement by free iliac bone grafts are largely similar to those used in primary bone grafting following resection of benign tumors (Fig. 2).

Rehabilitation of Masticatory Function

Masticatory function is not restored by means of bony mandibular replacement alone; its restoration requires further measures. For some years now, we have been using a new method in the rehabilitation of masticatory function: dental replacement fixed to enosseous implants. Critical evaluation of the so-called preprosthetical surgical measure to improve the denture-bearing site following reconstruction of the jaws has given unsatisfying results. In contrast, basic research and clinical long-term studies have produced favorable data on the feasibility and chances of success of enosseous implants used to stabilize dental replacement following mandibular reconstruction (Neukam et al. 1987, 1989, 1990).

In free bone grafts, enosseous implants may be inserted secondarily after bony remodeling of the graft has been completed. The implants serve as abutments for the dental replacement. In general, the implants are inserted at the same time as the osteosynthetic material is removed, i.e., 4–6 months after bone grafting. At this time, the surface of free bone grafts that have been taken without complications already consists of strong cortical bone.

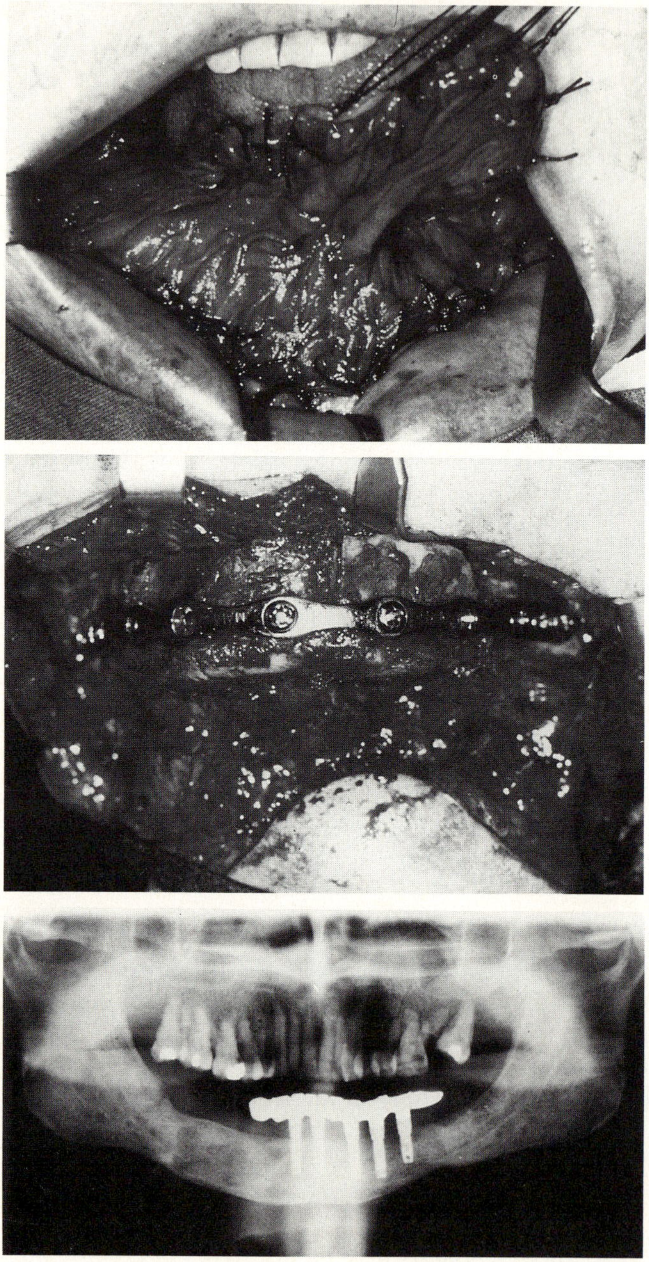

a

b

c

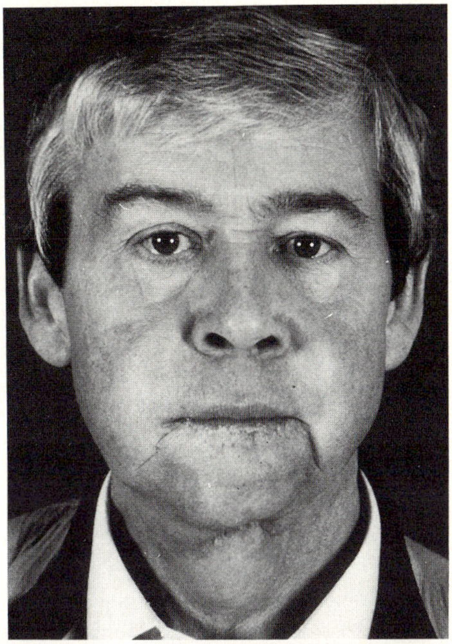

d

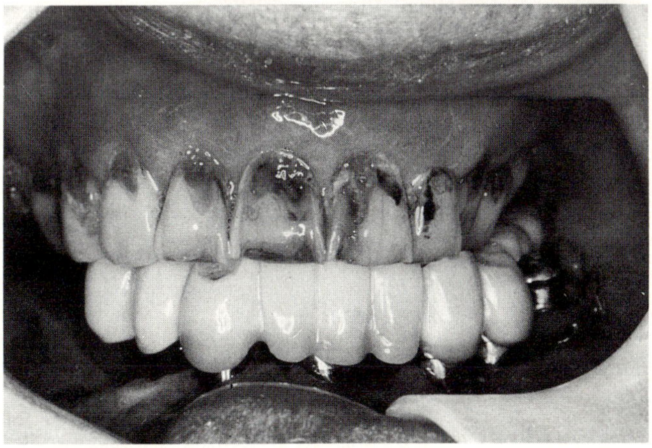

e

Fig. 2a–e. Microvascular jejunal graft and secondary reconstruction of the mandible with a free bone transplant in a 60-year-old patient. **a** After preoperative radiation (32 Gy), a hemimandibulectomy including the chin with resection of the right part of the floor of the mouth and the lateral and frontal aspect of the tongue was performed. The mandible was stabilized by a free rib bone graft, and the mucosal defect was primarily reconstructed by a microvascular revascularized jejunal graft. **b** Preparation of the free iliac bone graft for secondary mandibular osteoplasty 2 years after tumor resection fixed with a stable plate. **c** Radiographic findings 5 years after tumor resection and 2.5 years after rehabilitation with a prosthesis anchored to implants. **d** The extraoral aspect shows the contour of the chin and the lateral parts of the mandible. **e** The removable denture on the implants piercing the jejunal graft

The surgical techniques used for implantation following previous bone grafting are similar to those applied when inserting implants into atrophic jaws. They are covered and left to be taken by the recipient bone for 3–6 months. After this healing phase, they are exposed and may be loaded by carrying dental replacements.

In recent years, we have provided more than 50 patients with implants following bone grafting. The clinical results have shown that the resorption rate of bone grafts adequately loaded by enosseous, osseointegrated implants is low. It is possible to restore masticatory function by the subsequent incorporation of bridgework. Implantations have also been successful in previously irradiated jaws (50 Gy) if performed at least 2 years after completion of radiotherapy.

In poor recipient sites following radiotherapy or previous wound infection, microvascular bone grafts are increasingly used for secondary reconstruction, since they have the advantage of an independent blood supply. In addition, they provide the possibility of simultaneously grafting soft tissue to the recipient site, thereby decisively improving the quality of the recipient site and replacing soft tissue. The disadvantages of microvascular bone grafts lie in the fact that, in large extensive defects, the possibilities of contouring and adapting the microvascular graft are limited and the operation is further prolonged.

Since the vitality of microvascular bone grafts is maintained after grafting, insertion of implants into the graft at the time of grafting is possible. After a healing phase of 3–4 months, during which the implants, become covered with tissue, the implants are exposed when the plates are removed, and finally a denture carried by the implants is incorporated.

References

Cuono CB, Ariyan S (1980) Immediate reconstruction of a composite mandibular defect with a regional osteomusculocutaneous flap. Plast Reconstr Surg 65:477–485

Hausamen J-E, Neukam FW (1992) Transplantation von Knochen. In: Herberhold C (ed) Verhandlungsbericht 1992 der Deutschen Gesellschaft für Hals-Nasen-Ohren-Heilkunde, Kopf- und Hals-Chirurgie. Eur Arch Oto Rhino Laryngol, pp 163–177

Lexer E (1908) Die Verwendung der freien Knochenplastik nebst Versuchen über Gelenkversteifung und Gelenktransplantation. Langenbecks Arch Chir 86:939–954

Neukam FW, Hausamen J-E, Scheller H, Feldmann G (1987) Knochentransplantation in Kombination mit enossalen Implantaten. In: Kastenbauer E, Wilmes E, Mees K (eds) Das Transplantat in der plastischen Chirurgie. Sasse, Rotenburg-Wümme, pp 41–44

Neukam FW, Hausamen J-E, Scheller H (1989) Functional and esthetic rehabilitation with Branemark implants following oncologic surgery. In: Albrektson T, Zarb GA (eds) The Branemark osseointegrated implant. Quintessence, Chicago, pp 147–162

Neukam FW, Schmelzeisen R, Reilmann L, Kärcher H, Bothe K, Scheller H (1990)

Plastisch-rekonstruktive Maßnahmen mit freien mikrovaskulären Knochentransplantaten in Kombination mit Implantaten. Fortschr Kiefer Gesichtschir 35:79–82

Rehrmann A (1955) Kinnaufbau mit prothesenfähigem knöchernen Kieferbogen. Dtsch Zahn Mund Kieferheilkd 21:433–445

Rehrmann A (1978) Das freie Knochentransplantat zum Unterkieferersatz unter besonderer Berücksichtigung der Kinnrekonstruktion. Fortschr Kiefer Gesichtschir 23:39–43

Reichenbach E, Schönberger A (1957) 50 Jahre Knochentransplantate. Dtsch Zahn Mund Kieferheilkd 26:436–445

Reuther J, Steinau U (1980) Mikrochirurgische Dünndarmtransplantation zur Rekonstruktion großer Tumordefekte der Mundhöhle. Z Mund Kiefer Gesichtschir 4:131–136

Riediger D (1988) Restoration of masticatory function by microsurgically revascularized iliac crest bone grafts using enosseous implants. Plast Reconstr Surg 81:861–877

Riediger D, Büsing CM, D'Hoedt B, Pielsticker W (1986) Knochentransplantat mit mikrovaskulärem Anschluß als Implantatbett für enossale Implantate. Dtsch Zahnarztl Z 41:989–992

Salibian AH, Rappaport I, Furnas DW, Achauer BM (1985) Microvascular reconstruction of the mandible. Am J Surg 140:499–502

Taylor GI, Miller GDH, Ham FJ (1975) The free vascularized bone graft. A clinical extension of microvascular techniques. Plast Reconstr Surg 55:533–544

Taylor GI, Townsend P, Corlett R (1979) Superiority of the deep circumflex iliac vessels as a supply for free groin flaps. Clinical work. Plast Reconstr Surg 64:745–759

Surgery of Oropharyngeal Cancer

C. von Ilberg

Zentrum für Hals-Nasen-Ohrenheilkunde, Klinikum der Johann-Wolfgang-Goethe-Universität, Theodor-Stern-Kai 7, 60596 Frankfurt am Main, Germany

In recent years we have observed an increasing number of head and neck malignancies with the primary lesion in the oropharynx (Bettinger et al. 1991). The main locations are the tonsils, the base of the tongue, the soft palate, and the pharyngeal wall (Table 1).

In the surgery of these tumors it is important to have a maximum operating field over this complicated area. The usual surgical approaches are via the following: transoral, median mandibulotomy, lateral mandibulotomy, partial mandibulectomy, lateral pharyngotomy, and anterior pharyngotomy. The surgical procedure consists of three separate steps: (1) resection of the primary tumor, (2) surgery of the regional lymph nodes, and (3) reconstruction.

There is a high incidence of lymph node involvement in oropharynx cancer (Table 2). Surgery of the lymph nodes is, therefore, of particular importance. As about 50% of our T1 tumors already show signs of N1 disease, we consider an elective homolateral neck dissection to be necessary, even in the early stages of disease. In cases in which tumor invasion of the lymph nodes is detected by histological examination, a contralateral neck dissection is recommended. Our aim is to preserve the sternocleidomastoid muscle and the 11th cranial nerve unless these structures have been infiltrated by the tumor. Irrespective of the fact that neck dissection is a standard operation – frequently carried out by residents – it requires great

Table 1. Local distribution of oropharynx cancer

Location	Occurrence (%)
Tonsils	52
Base of tongue	31
Soft palate	14
Dorsal wall	3

Table 2. Involvement of lymph nodes in oropharynx cancer

Type of node[a]	Incidence (%)
N0	29
N1	58
N2	7
N3	7
N1–3	72

[a] Tumor Node Metastasis (TNM) classification

responsibility and precision because a high proportion of recurrences appear at the upper neck dissection region.

As far as the resection of the primary tumor is concerned, the importance of resection in healthy tissue must be pointed out. In serial sections of tumor specimens, we were able to clearly demonstrate the correlation between resection in healthy versus infiltrated tissue and the survival time of the patients (Fig. 1). On the other hand, resection in infiltrated tissue is clearly related to the tumor stage (Table 3). Resection in healthy tissue may turn out to be difficult for several reasons: deep infiltration of the tumor, sub-

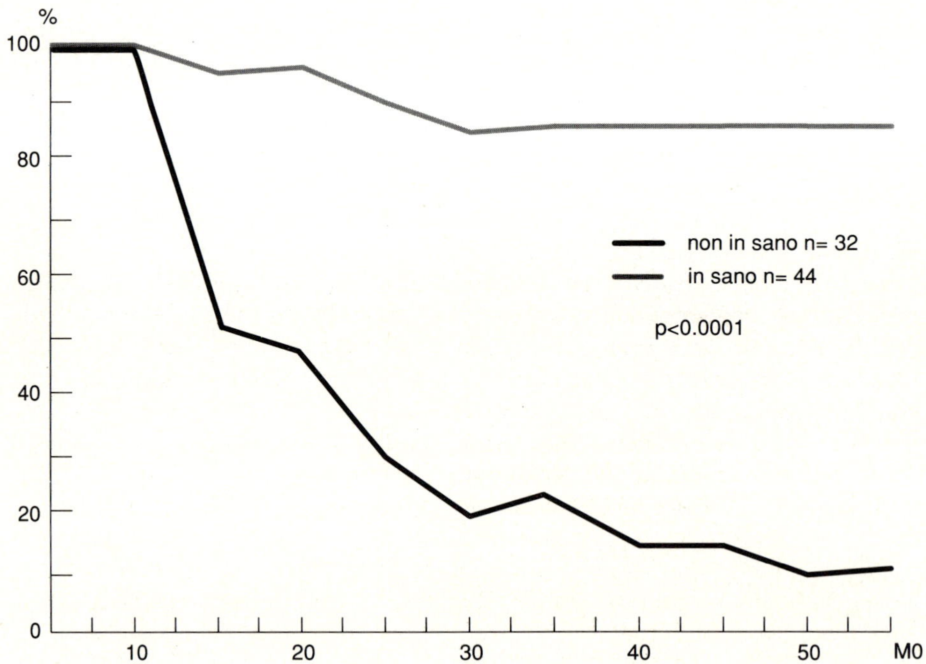

Fig. 1. Survival time of patients ($n = 76$) after resection in sano versus non insano (Bettinger et al. 1991)

Table 3. Histological results of resection

Tumor	*n*	in sano		non insano	
		n	%	*n*	%
T1	28	26	92.9	2	7.1
T2	30	25	83.3	5	16.7
T3	32	22	68.8	10	31.3
T4	39	23	59.0	16	41.0
Total	129	96		33	

mucous growth of the primary lesion, and/or the unsatisfactory visibility of the inferior resection border where the surgical access is inadequate. This explains why we find most insufficient resection borders at the lower base of the tongue, which in some cases is difficult to expose properly. The rate of resection in infiltrated tissue is even higher in cases following preoperative radio- or chemotherapy, because of the invisible tumor margins. Limited lesions (T1, T2) can be resected by the transoral access using a CO_2 laser or a high-frequency knife. Here again we see a high risk of inadequate resection in cases with deep infiltration. More advanced lesions (T3, T4) should be operated via exterior access route. The handling of the mandible is one of the crucial problems in oropharynx carcinoma. This is especially the case in carcinoma of the tonsil, which shows a particular tendency to infiltrate towards the mandible. In many cases of advanced carcinoma of the tonsils, we have to resect parts of the mandible for oncological reasons to ensure enbloc resection. Lateral pharyngotomy provides adequate access to the lower lateral oropharynx when the hypopharynx, the inferior base of the tongue, and/or the larynx are involved.

Different problems arise in the reconstruction of surgical damage after resection of oropharynx cancer. Minor lesions of the tongue, tonsils, or soft palate – particularly after laser surgery – do not require any reconstruction. Damage measuring up to 3 cm will heal spontaneously within a matter of weeks by self-repairing growth of the mucosa. T1 and T2 lesions usually can, and should, be covered by free grafts or local mucosa flaps without difficulty. T3 and T4 defects with a diameter of more than 4 cm require more sophisticated reconstruction techniques. As it would be impossible to mention even only all the most frequently used methods, I will concentrate on three techniques which have turned out to be most reliable in oropharynx reconstruction: (1) the pectoralis major musculocutaneous flap (Aryan 1979), (2) the myofascial flap, and (3) the free microvascular jejunum graft. The advantages and disadvantages of these three techniques are shown in Table 4. Any major surgery of the oropharynx is accompanied by preliminary tracheostomy. The different techniques used to reconstruct the mandible after mandibulotomy or partial mandibulectomy are dealt with in the chap-

Table 4. Oropharynx reconstruction techniques

Technique	Advantage	Disadvantage
Myocutaneous flap	Easy technique High success rate	Cosmetic problems Hair growth at donor site
Myofascial flap	Mucosa covering No skin damage at donor site	Thin fascia Occasional healing problems
Free jejunum graft	High quality mucosa Short recovery time Good functional results	Extended operation time

ter by Hausamen and Neukam and will not be discussed here, although I would like to point out that reconstruction of the resected mandible is not indicated in every case. Particularly in advanced carcinoma with high-dose preoperative radiotherapy, the reconstructive procedures seem to be problematic or even contraindicated. In these cases, prosthetic aids can be a good substitute for the function of the mandible.

Finally, we should point out that in cases of extended resection and reconstructive surgery of the oropharynx, various functional problems may arise. Two major problems should be addressed:

1. The larger the reconstructed area in the course of tumor resection, the greater the functional problems following surgery – such as swallowing disorders and aspiration – usually are. The reasons for the functional problems are the impaired soft palate structure, the dysfunction of the ninth, tenth, and 12th cranial nerve, the lack of muscular function of the transplant, and finally the formation of a sphincter-like stenotic ring at the esophagus entrance (Okamura et al. 1992). Consequently, these patients suffer from long-lasting swallowing disorders which require elaborated training programs. For these patients, we started a diagnostic and training program based on exterior pressure measurements during the swallowing process, which are analyzed by a computer program. With the same program the functional progress during the recovery phase can be monitored (Müller et al. 1992).
2. As was pointed out earlier, we have to keep in mind that prognosis of disease rapidly decreases with the increase of tumor size. Therefore, we must be aware that in extremely advanced tumor stages, our surgery acquires a more and more palliative character.

References

Ariyan S (1979) The pectoralis major myocutaneous falp: a versatile flap for reconstruction in the head and neck. Plast Reconstr Surg 63:73–81

Bettinger R, Loerz M, von Ilberg C, Desloovere C (1991) Histologisch kontrollierte Tumorchirurgie: Pathohistologische und immunhistochemische Untersuchungen zur Operationsradikalität bei Plattenepithelkarzinomen des HNO-Bereiches. Otorhinolaryngol Nova 1:140–145

Müller C, Roitman R, Yarkony S (1992) Diagnostik und Therapieverfahren bei Schluckstörungen mit Hilfe eines Kehlkopfbewegungsmessers und Trainingsprogramm einer interdisziplinären Arbeitsgruppe. Vortrag Deutsche Gesellschaft für Phoniatrie und Pädaudiologie, Garmisch-Partenkirchen

Okamura H, Inaki S, Mori T (1991) Swallowing function following hypopharyngeal reconstruction with the pectoralis major musculocutaneous flap. Auris Nasus Larynx 18:383–389

Surgical Management of Cervical Lymph Nodes in Patients with Oral and Oropharyngeal Cancer

G.B. Snow, M.W.M. van den Brekel, C.R. Leemans, and P. Patel

Department of Otolaryngology/Head and Neck Surgery, Free University Hospital, de Boelelaan 1117, 1081 HV Amsterdam, The Netherlands

Introduction

The incidence of neck metastases in oral cancer is approximately 50%, whereas cancers arising in the oropharynx have a metastatic rate of well over 50%. In general, it holds true that the more advanced the primary tumour, the higher the incidence of cervical metastases. The distribution of lymphatic metastases is, for the most part, explicable in mechanical and anatomical terms (Lindberg 1972; Shah 1990; Shah et al. 1990; Candela et al. 1990). The filter and barrier function of lymph nodes appears to be effective in the initial stage, as lymphatic spread is generally limited initially to the first echelon of lymph nodes.

It is well recognized that the status of the cervical lymph nodes is the single most important prognostic factor in squamous cell carcinoma of the head and neck. When nodal metastases exist at presentation or develop subsequently, cure rates decrease roughly by 50% (Spiro et al. 1974). To date, clinical assessment of the status of cervical lymph nodes has not been very accurate, although newer imaging techniques are being introduced; these are discussed below. In view of the inaccuracy of clinical assessment of the status of neck nodes, it is not surprising that retrospective clinicopathological analyses of large series of patients who had undergone neck dissections have demonstrated that histological parameters of neck node metastases are much more reliable than clinical parameters. This emphasizes the importance of neck dissection as a staging procedure, apart from its therapeutic effect. Extranodal spread and the number of positive nodes are the two histological factors that are of most prognostic significance as to the risk of recurrence in the neck (Cachin et al. 1979; Snow et al. 1986). The number of histologically positive nodes (more than three), extranodal spread, and lymph node metastases at multiple levels in the neck have also been shown to be prognostically significant for the risk of distant metastases (Leemans et al. 1992; Vikram et al. 1984).

Table 1. UICC TNM classification for lymph node metastases

Code	Type of node
Nx	Regional lymph nodes cannot be assessed
N0	No regional lymph node metastases
N1	Single ipsilateral node 3 cm or less in diameter
N2a	Single ipsilateral node more than 3 cm, but not more than 6 cm, in diameter
N2b	Multiple ipsilateral lymph nodes none more than 6 cm in diameter
N2c	Bilateral or contralateral lymph nodes, none more than 6 cm in diameter
N3	Lymph node more than 6 cm in diameter

Assessment of Cervical Lymph Node Metastases

For an appropriate, definitive treatment to be planned for any cancer in the oral cavity and oropharynx, it is of utmost importance to determine the status of the cervical lymph nodes in the neck. The UICC TNM classification (Hermanek and Sobin 1987) defines the regional lymph node (N) categories as shown in Table 1. Although clinical palpation of the neck is still widely used for staging of the neck, it is generally accepted that this is not very accurate. More recently, computed tomography (CT), magnetic resonance imaging (MRI), ultrasound (US) and US-guided fine needle aspiration cytology (FNAC) have also been used in an effort to improve the results of clinical staging.

Clinical Palpation

The location, consistency, and size of a lymph node as well as the type of neck and the experience of the examiner determine whether a lymph node is clinically palpable. In experienced hands, nodes as small as 0.5 cm can be detected in superficial areas such as the submandibular area and as small as 1.0 cm in deeper areas such as the subdigastric tissues (Sako et al. 1964). Micrometastases can occur in nodes smaller than these, giving rise to false negative results that may be in the order of 20%–30% (Ali et al. 1985). Similarly, normal nodes may vary in size, the largest being 2.0 cm (Hibbert et al. 1983), and can be readily palpable. Thus, clinical palpation can give rise to false positive results in up to 20% of cases (Ali et al. 1985). Clearly, if treatment plans and prognostic information are to be based on staging of neck nodes, then an improvement is desirable in both sensitivity (so that patients who require treatment to the neck are selected to receive it) and specificity (so that patients who do not require treatment to the neck are spared the unnecessary treatment and morbidity).

Computed Tomography

The introduction of high-resolution CT scans brought with it the hope and potential for detecting "occult" (not clinically palpable) metastases. There are, however, conflicting reports in the literature as to the value of routine CT scanning for staging of neck nodes. In a retrospective study, Feinmesser et al. (1987) from Toronto showed similar sensitivity rates for clinical examination and CT scanning (61.5% and 59.6%, respectively). The false positive rate for clinical examination was 8.6%, compared to 18.4% for CT. They therefore concluded that CT offers no advantage over physical examination in staging neck nodes. Others have shown that CT scanning has a higher sensitivity in detecting metastatic disease than physical examination (Friedman et al. 1984; Mancuso et al. 1981, 1983; Stern et al. 1990; Stevens et al. 1985). The radiological criteria used for diagnosing a lymph node as malignant need to be considered. They include nodal size, central necrosis, pericapsular extentions, and obliteration of perivascular fat planes (Friedman et al. 1984; Mancuso et al. 1981, 1983). Using these criteria, Friedman et al. (1990b) reported a significantly greater sensitivity of the CT scan (87.1%) compared to clinical examination (72.3%). CT scanning would, therefore, seem appropriate in patients at high risk for metastases and those with a clinically palpable node to evaluate the contralateral neck.

Magnetic Resonance Imaging

MRI has better soft tissue contrast resolution than CT, and studies are now being reported on the efficacy of MRI with regard to staging of neck nodes. In a report based on 30 neck dissections in 27 patients, Feinmesser et al. (1990) showed that there was little advantage in using MRI over clinical examination in detection of cervical metastases. Their findings are in contrast to other reports including a recent large prospective study reported from the Free University Hospital, Amsterdam (van den Brekel et al. 1991a; Friedman et al. 1990a). It should be noted, however, that reliable comparison of sensitivity and specificity reported in different series is difficult due to different patient populations and particularly due to the varying radiological criteria and differing imaging techniques employed. More accurate criteria for cervical lymph node malignancy have been reported based on a pathoanatomical study by van den Brekel et al. (1990). Criteria for malignancy on MRI include: (a) evidence of central necrosis, (b) minimal axial diameter greater than 11 mm in the subdigastric area or greater than 10 mm in other areas, and (c) grouping of three or more borderline nodes (minimal axial diameter 1–2 mm less than above) in the lymph node draining region of the tumor. With these criteria, van den Brekel reported the sensitivity and specificity of MRI to be 81% and 88%, respectively (overall error, 16%), as compared with 68% and 67%, respectively, for clinical examination (overall error, 32%). In the clinically N0 neck (see Table 1), the MRI sensitivity and specificity were 60% and 89%, respectively. These results indicate that contrast-enhanced MRI can be a valuable tool for cervical lymph node staging, with the overall error being half that of clinical palpation. As only 60% of the clinically occult metastases can be detected by MRI, one cannot rely exclusively on MRI findings. It can, however, be used in conjunction with such other factors as the size, site, and histological grading of the primary tumor for selection of patients for prophylactic treatment of the neck.

Ultrasound and Ultrasound-Guided Fine Needle Aspiration Cytology

There have been numerous reports on the use of US and US-guided FNAC in recent years (Baatenburg de Jong et al. 1988, 1989; van den Brekel et al. 1990, 1991b; Bruneton and Normand 1987; Bruneton et al. 1984; Hajec et al. 1986). US does not allow differentiation between enlarged lymph nodes and enlarged metastatic nodes (Baatenburg de Jong et al. 1989; van den Brekel et al. 1991b). The criteria suggested for such differentiation are size (minimal axial diameter) and grouping of more than three borderline lymph nodes (van den Brekel et al. 1990). Sensitivity for the detection of nodes can be increased for all imaging techniques by using stricter criteria (such as a smaller minimal axial diameter), but this inevitably results in a decreased specificity for metastatic disease (Baatenburg de Jong et al. 1989; van den Brekel et al. 1991b). The advantage of US is that with the addition of US-guided FNAC, the specificity, too, can be improved (Baatenburg de Jong et al. 1989; van den Brekel et al. 1991b). Thus, US-guided FNAC was shown to have a sensitivity of 76% and a specificity of 100% (accuracy of 89%) in necks that were clinically negative by palpation alone (van den Brekel et al. 1991b). These results are an improvement on those reported in the literature for CT and MRI (van den Brekel et al. 1991a; Friedman et al. 1984; Friedman et al. 1990b; Stern et al. 1990) and are of great importance in enabling the detection of occult metastatic disease in the neck.

US-guided FNAC is a technique requiring both expertise and experience which is not presently available in the majority of medical centers. It is highly recommended that routine CT or MRI scanning of the neck be employed in all patients with oral and oropharyngeal cancer, as well as in those with advanced cancer posteriorly in the oral cavity, who already require CT or MRI for the assessment of the primary tumor and can then have their necks evaluated at the same time without significant additional costs. Where expertise is available, US-guided FNAC should be used when the results of the other modalities are doubtful.

Surgical Management

Surgical Classification of Neck Dissections

Before discussing in detail the options for treatment of lymph node metastases in the neck, the terminology used will be clearly defined. The need for standardization of neck dissection terminology has been recognized for

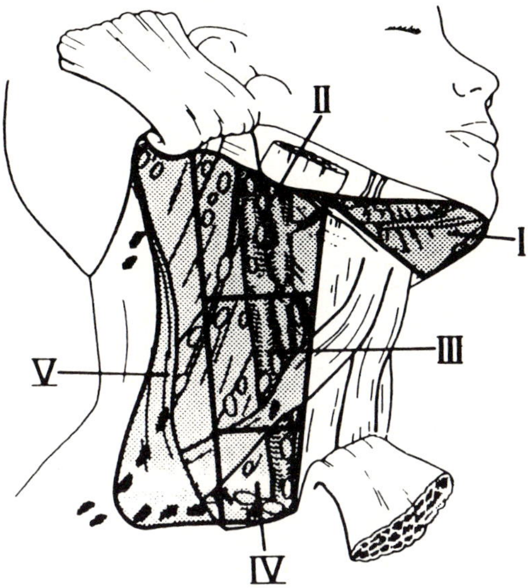

Fig. 1. The level system for describing the location of lymph nodes in the neck. *Level I* indicates the submental and submandibular group of nodes; *level II*, the upper jugular group; *level III*, the middle jugular group; *level IV*, the lower jugular group; *level V*, the posterior triangle (occipital) group

some time. The Committee of Head and Neck Surgery and Oncology of the American Academy of Otolaryngology and Head and Neck Surgery in the United States have produced an "official" report for standardizing neck dissection terminology, and it is this version which is adopted here (Robbins et al. 1991).

Figure 1 is an artist's depiction of the anatomical groups of cervical nodes. Level I contains the submental and submandibular groups of nodes, levels II–IV the jugular nodes, and level V the posterior or occipital nodes. The classical radical neck dissection (RND) is the standard procedure removing all levels of cervical nodes (levels I – V), including the sternomastoid muscle, the internal jugular vein, and the accessory nerve. The modified RND is an alternative to the RND and involves the preservation of one or more nonlymphatic structures (accessory nerve, internal jugular vein, and sternomastoid muscle). In the selective neck dissection, there is preservation of one or more lymph node groups routinely removed in the RND. The accessory nerve, internal jugular vein, and the sternomastoid muscle are usually preserved. The commonly performed procedures include the supraomohyoid dissection, in which levels I, II, and III are excised, and the anterolateral neck dissection, in which levels I, II, III, and IV are removed. Finally, the extended RND involves removal of additional lymph node groups or nonlymphatic structures relative to RND.

Management of cervical lymph nodes can be considered as either *elective* (when there is no clinical evidence of lymph node involvement) or *therapeutic* (when lymph nodes are clinically involved with tumor).

Elective Neck Dissection

The rationale for elective treatment of the neck is based on the following premises. Firstly, it appears that occult disease in the neck will inevitably develop into clinically manifest disease, as the incidence of histologically tumor-positive nodes in elective neck dissection specimens corresponds closely to the nodal conversion rate during follow-up of patients initially staged as N0, whose necks were not treated. Secondly, it is well known that despite close regular follow-up, some patients will develop inoperable disease in the neck if a "wait and see" policy is pursued. Finally, untreated occult disease in cervical lymph nodes may predispose the patient to developing distant metastases while the lymph node is growing to a clinically detectable size. This is supported by the observation that the larger the amount of disease in the neck, the higher the incidence of distant metastases, whereas distant metastases are rare in patients who have never developed lymph node metastases (Merino et al. 1977; Snow et al. 1986). The arguments against elective treatment of cervical lymph nodes are as follows: if the risk of occult metastases is low, then one is subjecting a large proportion of patients to a treatment that they do not require. Such treatment may also remove or destroy a barrier to cancer spread, which may be particularly important if recurrence at the primary site should occur at a later date. Opponents of elective treatment also point to the morbidity and mortality associated with elective surgical treatment, although this is slight with the modified types of neck dissection currently in use.

In general, elective treatment of the neck is considered to be indicated clinically when there is a high likelihood of occult nodal metastases, when the status of the cervical lymph nodes cannot be adequately assessed, when the patient will be unavailable for regular follow-up, or when the neck needs to be entered for surgical access and treatment of the primary tumor. Unfortunately, reliable practical predictors of the risk of occult metastases are not available. Although the T stage of the primary tumor has been reported by Mendenhall's group (Mendenhall et al. 1980) to be related to the incidence of occult metastases, other investigators, such as Ali et al. (1985), have been unable to confirm any such relationship. There is, however, strong evidence for a relationship between tumor thickness and regional node involvement (Spiro et al. 1986). The presence of microvascular involvement in the immediate vicinity of the primary tumor appears to be highly predictive of involvement of regional nodes (Close et al. 1987), although such invasion is difficult to detect in biopsy material.

In general, a frequency of occult metastases exceeding 15%–20% is considered to be sufficient to justify elective treatment of the neck nodes. Most sites and stages of squamous cell carcinoma in the oral cavity and oropharynx qualify for elective treatment on this basis. There is good evidence that elective irradiation of the neck is as effective as elective surgical treatment (Chow et al. 1989). The choice is therefore influenced by the mode of treatment of the primary tumor: if the primary tumor is treated by surgery, the neck is also treated surgically, whereas the neck will be treated by radiotherapy when the primary tumor is irradiated.

In actual practice, the classical RND has only a limited role in the elective treatment of the neck. The choice in most cases, therefore, lies between a modified RND or a selective neck dissection. The modified RNDs are well-established procedures and have stood the test of time.

Selective neck dissections have been introduced relatively recently. The rationale for selective neck dissections is that only those groups of lymph nodes need to be removed which, on the basis of the site of the primary tumor, are at highest risk of containing metastases (Lindberg 1972; Shah 1990). The supraomohyoid is the most commonly performed type of selective neck dissection, particularly in cases of anterior tongue and anterior floor of mouth cancers. It is appropriate that some comments should be made with regard to both the indications and the technique for this procedure.

There have been recent trends to extend the indications for a specific type of selective neck dissection to primary sites other than that for which the procedure was originally intended. Thus, the supraomohyoid neck dissection, which is primarily designed for the elective treatment of the neck in anterior tongue and anterior floor of mouth cancers, is increasingly used in managing cancers of the oropharynx (Medina and Byers 1989; Spiro et al. 1988). Until more long-term results are available for this operation, it is recommended that the indications for supraomohyoid neck dissection be limited to anterior tongue and anterior floor of mouth cancers. It is also felt that lymph nodes in level IV should also be included, thus extending the supraomohyoid procedure to a proper anterolateral dissection (levels I, II, III, and IV). Furthermore, the anterolateral dissection in our institution is carried out only when bilateral neck dissections are indicated (for example, when these tumors are located in or close to the midline), a modified RND being preferred for unilateral treatment.

With regard to technique, selective neck dissection can be technically more demanding and requires greater surgical experience. The posterior limit of such an anterolateral neck dissection is also difficult to define surgically, and it is particularly important to dissect free the accessory nerve in its upper course and remove all the fibroadipose tissue containing lymph nodes from the upper posterior part of level II.

Frozen section examination of suspicious lymph nodes perioperatively may allow extension of the selective procedure into a modified RND if the node is proved positive. In some hospital centers, such as the Gustave Roussy Institute near Paris, it is usual practice to send the whole specimen for frozen section. Although this appears to be a logical approach, it is obviously quite time-consuming and not always practical in many institutions. Some surgeons, such as Spiro et al. (1988), would rather rely on postoperative radiotherapy if microscopic nodal involvement is reported at routine paraffin section examination.

Therapeutic Neck Dissection

The choice of surgical procedure lies between the classical RND and a form of modified RND, although some clinicians, such as Medina and Byers (1989), advocate selective neck dissection for N1 disease (see Table 1). The classical RND as described by Crile in 1906 is still comonly in use in many centers for the treatment of clinically evident lymphatic neck metastases. Over the last two decades, however, modified RNDs are increasingly being used in order to try to reduce the morbidity associated with classical RNDs (Schuller et al. 1983), but without compromising the efficacy of treatment. Compelling arguments and data in support of such a move are provided by a number of publications (Bocca and Pignataro 1967; Bocca et al. 1984; Dayal and da Silva 1971; Lingeman et al. 1977; Schuller et al. 1983).

Structures that may be preserved in a modified RND include the accessory nerve, the internal jugular vein, and the sternomastoid muscle. The internal jugular vein has a close relationship to some of the most frequently involved groups of nodes in the neck (levels II, III, and IV). One therefore needs to be very cautious with regard to advocating its preservation, although we recommend that it should be preserved on the least involved side in cases of bilateral neck dissections in order to prevent the serious sequelae of bilateral venous obstruction.

Preservation of the sternomastoid muscle makes the dissection more difficult and possibly less radical in the upper neck, whereas the advantage of preserving a more normal contour of the neck is perhaps not of great importance in the usually elderly male patient. In our experience, preservation of the sternomastoid muscle in the node-positive neck has not been justified.

The question remains as to whether the accessory nerve should be preserved, particularly as the most disabling morbidity of the classical neck dissection is the so-called frozen shoulder syndrome. Carenfelt and Eliasson (1981) have confirmed that the accessory nerve may indeed be preserved without jeopardizing the chances of cure in selected therapeutic neck dissections, and this is consistent with our own experience. However, it has been clearly demonstrated that metastases are not uncommon along the superior portion of the nerve, particularly in cancer of the oropharynx and posterior oral cavity, so that the feasibility of preservation of the accessory nerve in each individual case has to be carefully evaluated by the surgeon during the actual dissection. It should be remembered that preservation of the nerve does not preclude impaired shoulder function (Carenfelt and Eliasson 1981) and that physical therapy rehabilitaton programs can minimize shoulder problems in some patients in whom the nerve has had to be sacrificed.

Postoperative Radiotherapy

When extranodal spread and/or multiple positive nodes are present in the neck dissection specimen, there is a high risk of recurrence in the neck (Snow et al. 1982). It has been demonstrated that in these circumstances, postoperative radiotherapy is capable of reducing the recurrence rate in the neck considerably (Bartelink et al. 1983; Leemans et al. 1990; Snow et al. 1986). As a consequence, it is our usual practice today to give postoperative radiotherapy when the previously mentioned unfavorable histological factors are reported by the pathologist.

Results of Treatment

The efficacy of any form of treatment to the cervical lymph nodes is reflected in the regional control rate after such treatment. Although various studies report on the results of treatment to the cervical lymph nodes, it is important to recognize that valid comparisons are often difficult due to differences in tumor and patient populations and types of neck dissections carried out. Most series also often fail to take into account the influence that recurrence at the primary site may have on regional control rates by causing reseeding in the neck. Uniform nomenclature and classification of neck dissections, inclusion of histological status of lymph nodes in surgical series, and standardization of indications for postoperative radiotherapy should all help in the reporting of comparable results.

The regional recurrence rate after surgical treatment of the neck in patients with head and neck cancer correlates well with the histopathological involvement of the neck and whether postoperative radiotherapy is used. If patients with recurrence at the primary site are excluded from analysis, the regional recurrence rate for the histopathologically tumor-positive neck is approximately 10% (Leemans et al. 1990; Mantravadi et al. 1983; Molinari et al. 1980) and for histologically negative necks 3% (Leemans et al. 1990). With a policy of giving postoperative radiotherapy to patients with either more than two histologically positive nodes, or those with extranodal spread, Leemans et al. (1990) showed that these patients fared no worse than those with one or two histologically positive nodes and no extranodal spread (and no postoperative radiotherapy). They all had a regional recurrence rate of around 10%. This testifies to the efficacy of postoperative radiotherapy and has led us to use routine radiotherapy for patients with two histologically positive nodes as well. Some clincians have advocated extending the indications to even include patients with only *one* histologically positive node without extranodal spread. It should be remembered, however, that any potential benefits for this group are likely to be limited to a few patients and need to be weighed against the morbidity of mucositis, xerostomia, and skin induration to many patients.

Conclusion

Surgical treatment of neck nodes provides valuable prognostic information about the status of the lymph nodes, which allows further treatment to be tailored to the needs of the patient. Not only can postoperative radiotherapy be planned rationally on the basis of histological results, but also patients at highest risk for distant metastases can possibly be identified for adjuvant systemic therapy such as chemotherapy or immunotherapy. The value of such treatment has yet to be established, and any such treatment should therefore be part of a well-designed prospective randomized trial whenever possible.

Elective treatment of the neck is thought to be indicated if the risk of occult metastatic nodes is judged to be greater than 15%–20% (Ali et al. 1985; Lee and Krause 1975; Ogura et al. 1971). If techniques such as US-guided FNAC can be used to identify three out of four patients with occult nodes (van den Brekel et al. 1991b), the risk of undetected metastases can be improved from approximately 30% to 7.5% in a group of patients previously staged as N0 by clinical palpation alone. The implications of this in terms of avoiding elective surgery are obvious. However, it should be remembered that techniques such as US-guided FNAC are technically demanding and results from medical centers experienced in this procedure cannot be generally applied. It must, therefore, be emphasized that each institution intending to use such a technique to help modify existing treatment strategy would first need to verify the accuracy of the procedure in its own hands. It is perhaps ironic that as more selective and less radical surgical procedures are being advocated for elective treatment of the neck, the very need for such treatment may require reappraisal in the light of advances in the accuracy of diagnostic procedures.

References

Ali S, Tiwari RM, Snow GB (1985) False positive and false negative neck nodes. Head Neck Surg 8:78–82

Baatenburg de Jong RJ, Rongen RJ, Jong PC de, Lameris JS, Knegt P (1988) Screening for lymph nodes in the neck with ultrasound. Clin Otolaryngol 13:5–9

Baatenburg de Jong RJ, Rongen RJ, Lameris JS, Harthoorn M, Verwoerd CDA,

Knegt P (1989) Metastatic neck disease: palpation vs ultrasound examination. Arch Otolaryngol Head Neck Surg 115:689–690
Bartelink H, Breur K, Hart G, Annyas AA, Slooten EA van, Snow GB (1983) The value of postoperative radiotherapy as an adjuvant to radical neck dissection. Cancer 52:1008–1013
Bocca E, Pignataro O (1967) A conservative technique in radical neck dissection. Ann Otol Rhinol Laryngol 76:975–988
Bocca E, Pignataro O, Oldini C, Cappa C (1984) Functional neck dissection: an evaluation and reviews of 843 cases. Laryngoscope 94:942–945
Bruneton JN, Normand F (1987) Cervical lymph nodes. In: Bruneton JN (ed) Ultrasonography of the neck. Springer, Berlin Heidelberg New York, pp 81–91
Bruneton JN, Roux P, Caramella E, Demard F, Vallicioni J, Chauvel P (1984) Ear, nose and throat cancer: ultrasound diagnosis of metastases to cervical lymph nodes. Radiology 152:771–773
Cachin Y, Sancho-Garnier H, Micheau C, Marandas P (1979) Nodal metastases from carcinomas of the oropharynx. Otolaryngol Clin North Am 12:145–154
Candela FC, Kotharai K, Shah JP (1990) Patterns of cervical lymph node metastases from squamous carcinoma of the oropharynx and hypopharynx. Head Neck 10:160–167
Carenfelt C, Eliasson K (1981) Radical neck dissection and permanent sequelae associated with spinal accessory nerve injuries. Acta Otolaryngol (Stockh) 91: 155–160
Chow JM, Levin BC, Krivit JS, Applebaum EA (1989) Radiotherapy or surgery for subclinical cervical node metastases. Arch Otolaryngol Head Neck Surg 115: 981–984
Close LG, Burns DK, Reisch J, Schaefer SD (1987) Microvascular invasion in cancer of the oral cavity and oropharynx. Arch Otolaryngol Head Neck Surg 113: 1191–1195
Crile G (1906) Excision of cancer of the head and neck with special reference to the plan of dissection based on 132 operations. JAMA 47:1780–1786
Dayal VS, da Silva AJ (1971) Functional and radical neck dissection. Arch Otolaryngol 93:413–415
Feinmesser R, Freeman JL, Noyek AM, Birt D (1987) Metastatic neck disease. A clinical/radiographic/pathologic correlative study. Arch Otolaryngol Head Neck Surg 113:1307–1310
Feinmesser R, Freeman JL, Noyek AM, Birt D, Gullane P, Mullen JB (1990) MRI and neck metastases: a clinical, radiological, pathological correlative study. J Otolaryngol 19:136–140
Friedman M, Shelton VK, Mafee M, Bellity P, Grybauskas V, Skolnik E (1984) Metastatic neck disease: evaluation by computed tomography. Arch Otolaryngol 110:443–447
Friedman M, Mafee MF, Pacella BL, Strorigl TL, Dew LL, Toriumi DM (1990a) Rationale for elective neck dissection in 1990. Laryngoscope 100:54–59
Friedman M, Toriumi DM, Mafee MF, Strorigl T (1990b) The role of computed tomographic scanning in evaluating the clinically negative neck. In: Fee WE, Goepfert H, Johns ME, Strong EW, Ward PH (eds) Head and neck cancer, vol 2. Decker, Toronto, pp 138–144
Hajec PC, Solomonowitz E, Turk R, Tscholakoff D, Kumpan W, Czembirek H (1986) Lymph nodes of the neck: evaluation with ultrasound. Radiology 158: 739–742
Hermanek P, Sobin LH (eds) (1987) TNM classification of malignant tumours. Springer, Berlin Heidelberg New York, p 14
Hibbert J, Marks NJ, Winter PJ, Shaheen OH (1983) Prognostic factors in oral

squamous cell carcinoma and their relation to clinical staging. Clin Otolaryngol 8:197–203

Lee JG, Krause CJ (1975) Radical neck dissection. Elective, therapeutic and secondary. Arch Otolaryngol 101:656–659

Leemans CR, Tiwari R, Waal I van der, Karim ABMF, Nauta JJP, Snow GB (1990) The efficacy of comprehensive neck dissection with or without postoperative radiotherapy in nodal metastases of squamous cell carcinoma of the upper respiratory and digestive tracts. Laryngoscope 100:1194–1198

Leemans CR, Tiwari R, Nauta JJP, Waal I van der, Snow GB (1992) Regional lymph node involvement and its significance in the development of distant metastases in head and neck carcinoma. Cancer (in press)

Lindberg RD (1972) Distribution of cervical lymph node metastases for squamous cell carcinoma of the upper respiratory tract. Cancer 29:1446–1449

Lingeman RE, Helmus C, Stephens R, Ulm J (1977) Neck dissection: radical or conservative. Ann Otol Rhinol Laryngol 86:737–744

Mancuso AA, Maceri D, Rice D, Hanafee W (1981) CT of cervical lymph node cancer. A J R 136:381–385

Mancuso AA, Harnsberger HR, Muraki AS, Stevens MH (1983) Computed tomography of cervical and retropharyngeal lymph nodes: normal anatomy, variants of normal, and applications in staging head and neck cancer: II. Pathology. Radiology 198:715–723

Mantravadi RVP, Skolnik EM, Haas RE, Applebaum EL (1983) Patterns of cancer recurrence in the postoperatively irradiated neck. Arch Otolaryngol 109:753–756

Medina JE, Byers RM (1989) Supraomohyoid neck dissection: rationale, indications, and surgical technique. Head Neck Surg 11:111–122

Mendenhall WM, Million RR, Cassisi NJ (1980) Elective neck irradiation in squamous cell carcinoma of the head and neck. Head Neck Surg 3:15–20

Merino OR, Lindberg RD, Fletcher GH (1977) An analysis of distant metastases from squamous cell carcinoma of the upper respiratory and digestive tracts. Cancer 40:145–151

Molinari R, Cantu G, Chiesa F, Grandi C (1980) Retrospective comparison of conservative and radical neck dissection in laryngeal cancer. Ann Otol Rhinol Laryngol 89:578–581

Ogura JH, Biller HF, Wette R (1971) Elective neck dissection for pharyngeal and laryngeal cancers: an evaluation. Ann Otol Rhinol Laryngol 80:646–651

Robbins KT, Medina JE, Wolfe GT, Levine PA, Sessions RB, Pruet CW (1991) Standardizing neck dissection terminology – official report of the Academy's Committee for Head and Neck Surgery and Oncology. Arch Otolaryngol Head Neck Surg 117:601–605

Sako K, Pradier RN, Marchetta FC, Pickren JW (1964) Fallibility of palpation in the diagnosis of metastases to the cervical nodes. Surg Gynecol Obstet 118:989–990

Schuller DE, Reiches NA, Hamaker RC, Lingeman RE, Weisberger EC, Suen JY, Conley JJ, Kelly DR, Miglets AW (1983) Analysis of disability resulting from treatment including radical neck dissection or modified neck dissection. Head Neck Surg 6:551–558

Shah JP (1990) Patterns of cervical lymph node metastases from squamous carcinoma of the upper aerodigestive tract. Am J Surg 160:405–409

Shah JP, Candela FC, Poddar AK (1990) The patterns of cervical lymph node metastases from squamous carcinoma of the oral cavity. Cancer 66:109–113

Snow GB, Annyas AA, van Slooten EA, Bartelink H, Hart AAM (1982) Prognostic factors of neck node metastasis. Clin Otolaryngol 7:185–192

Snow GB, Balm AJM, Arendse JW, Karim ABMF, Bartelink H, Waal I van der, Tiwari RM (1986) Prognostic factors in neck node metastases. In: Larson DL,

Ballantyne AJ, Guillamondegni OM (eds) Cancer in the neck. Evaluation and treatment. MacMillan, New York, pp 53–63
Spiro RH, Alfonso AE, Farr HW, Strong EW (1974) Cervical node metastases from epidermoid carcinoma of the oral cavity and oropharynx. A critical assessment of current staging. Am J Surg 128:562–567
Spiro RH, Huvos AG, Wong GY, Spiro JD, Gnecco CA, Strong EW (1986) Predictive value of tumour thickness in squamous carcinoma confined to the tongue and floor of the mouth. Am J Surg 152:345–350
Spiro JD, Spiro RH, Shah JP, Sessions RB, Strong EW (1988) Critical assessment of supraomohyoid neck dissection. Am J Surg 156:286–289
Stern WBR, Silver CE, Zeifer BA, Persky MS, Heller KS (1990) Computed tomography of the clinically negative neck. Head Neck 12:109–113
Stevens MH, Harnsberger HR, Mancuso AA, Davis RK, Johnson LP, Parkin JL (1985) Computed tomography of cervical lymph nodes: staging and management of head and neck cancer. Arch Otolaryngol 111:735–739
van den Brekel MWM, Stel HV, Castelijns JA, Nauta JJ, Waal I van der, Valk J, Meyer CJ, Snow GB (1990) Cervical lymph node metastases: assessment of radiologic criteria. Radiology 177:379–384
van den Brekel MWM, Castelijns JA, Croll GA, Stel HV, Valk J, Waal I van der, Golding RP, Meyer CJLM, Snow GB (1991a) Magnetic resonance imaging vs palpation of cervical lymph node metastases. Arch Otolaryngol Head Neck Surg 117:666–673
van den Brekel MWM, Castelijns JA, Stel HV, Luth WJ, Valk J, Waal I van der, Snow GB (1991b) Occult metastatic neck disease: detection with ultrasound and ultrasound-guided fine needle aspiration cytology. Radiology 180:457–461
Vikram B, Strong EW, Shah JP, Spiro R (1984) Failure at distant sites following mutimodality treatment for advanced head and neck cancer. Head Neck Surg 6:730–733

Radical Neck Dissection Versus Conservative Neck Dissection for Squamous Cell Carcinoma of the Oral Cavity

J. Bier[1]

Clinic for Maxillofacial Surgery, University Clinic Rudolf Virchow, Free University Berlin, Augustenburger Platz 1, 13344 Berlin, Germany

Introduction

The survival time of patients with squamous cell carcinoma of the oral cavity is similar to what it was 30 years ago. Despite more radical surgery, new chemotherapeutic agents, and improvements in radiotherapy, no significant changes have taken place. The 5-year survival rates vary between 37%, as stated by Byers (1985), and 51%, as stated by Ackermann et al. (1985). A survival rate of 41%–42% would appear to be more realistic, as shown by Platz and Hudec (1986) in two German-Austrian-Swiss Association for Head and Neck Tumors (DÖSAK) studies between 1952 and 1985 with a total of 2507 patients.

The lack of improvement in survival rates raises the question of whether we really need surgery as radical as that still being performed in many clinics.

For many years radical neck dissection has been a common procedure of operation for draining lymph nodes in patients with squamous cell carcinomas of the oral cavity. However, many attempts have been made to operate the draining lymph nodes in a more conservative way.

The Terminology of Neck Dissection

In connection with "radical" neck dissection – as described by Crile (1906) – terms such as "classical" "standard radical" "elective" "prophylactic" and "therapeutic" neck dissection are used. In connection with "conservative" neck dissection – as initially described by Bocca and Pignataro in 1967

---

[1] On behalf of the German-Austrian-Swiss Association for Head and NeckTumors (DÖSAK) within the German Society for Maxillofacial Surgery (DGMKG)

– terms such as "functional" neck dissection, already introduced 1 year before by Bocca (1966), "modified," "modified radical," "elective," and "prophylactic" neck dissection are used. The terms "suprahyoidal" and "supra-omohyoidal" neck dissection are also used. Later on, all these different terminologies of nonradical neck dissection were defined as "limited" neck dissection by O'Brien et al. (1987).

The multiplicity of all these different terms became even more confusing because the abbreviation CND was and still is used for "classical" as well as for "conservative" neck dissection.

The terms "elective" and "prophylactic" neck dissection are used for the No neck together with "radical" neck dissection, as described by Southwick et al. (1967) and by Kinsey and James (1962). The same terms are also used for "conservative" neck dissection, as described by Bocca et al. (1984) and O'Brien et al. (1987). The name "therapeutic" neck dissection, as described by Vandenbrough et al. (1980), has been used for the N+ neck together with "radical" neck dissection.

Because of this confusing terminology, an urgent demand for standardization was voiced in 1982 at a consensus conference of the DÖSAK (Bier 1982). As a result of this meeting, two terms have been defined and are now being used in the DÖSAK: "radical" and "conservative" neck dissection.

The surgical procedure of radical neck dissection has been defined according to the initial description by Crile (1906). The anatomical structures which have to be removed are:

1. Platysma, sternocleidomastoid muscle, omohyoid muscle, stylohyoid muscle, the distal part of the biventer cervicis, and the fascia colli
2. The accessory nerve, the descending branch of the hypoglossus nerve, and branches of the cervical plexus
3. The cervical vein, the superficial jugular vein, and the internal jugular vein
4. Fat tissue, the submandibular gland, and the lower part of the parotid gland.

Following these criteria, any variant of neck dissection leaving one of these structures in situ cannot be designated as "radical" neck dissection. The surgical procedure of "conservative" is similar to that of "radical" neck dissection. However, the platysma, the sternocleidomastoid muscle, the internal jugular vein, and the accessory nerve have to be left in place.

The necessity of a clear definition for the surgery of draining lymph nodes was also stated by Suen and Goefert (1987) and O'Brien et al. (1987). Therefore, a scheme was introduced in 1989 by Medina (Medina and Byers 1989) which has since been adopted by the American Academy of Otolaryngology. Three basic types of neck dissection are mentioned in this scheme: "comprehensive," "selective," and "extended" neck dissection. However, these three types are further divided into 11 subtypes. From a scientific point of view, this classification is well defined, but from a practical point of view it does not seem to be very useful.

Radical Neck Dissection Versus Conservative Neck Dissection

Comparing the literature of radical procedures with more conservative operations for the neck, the therapeutic results were controversial, and there was no prospective randomized clinical trial on this topic. Therefore, the DÖSAK started a study on this problem entitled "Radical neck dissection versus conservative neck dissection." The clinics listed in the Acknowledgements are involved in this ongoing clinical trial.

Patients and Treatment

Patients entering the study have to fulfil the following criteria:

1. Untreated squamous cell carcinoma of the oral cavity without metastases
2. Primary tumor on one side postcanine or postmolar, i.e., second or third part of the tongue, respectively
3. Nonpalpable or clinically negative, or clinically positive, movable lymph nodes in the neck

Group A is being treated with radical surgery at the primary tumor and radical neck dissection on the draining lymph nodes. Group B is also being treated with radical surgery at the primary, but conservative neck dissection for the draining lymph nodes.

On the ipsilateral tumor site, lymph nodes are treated by radical or conservative neck dissection and on the contralateral side, no therapy or suprahyoid neck dissection is performed. Patients are randomized according to the Treatment Dependent Prognostic Index (TPI) of the DÖSAK (Platz and Hudec 1986).

Surgery is the only treatment used in this study. However, the operation is followed by radiotherapy and/or chemotherapy in patients not operated on radically at the primary site and in patients with capsular rupture occurring in at least one lymph node. These patients are still in the study, but they are not evaluated.

Results

So far, 167 patients have been randomized and 104 patients are evaluable – 48 in group A and 56 in group B. The follow-up time is 456 days for group A and 463 days for group B. The mean age is 57 years – 59 years in group A and 55 years in group B. The sex distribution is 85% male and 15% female –

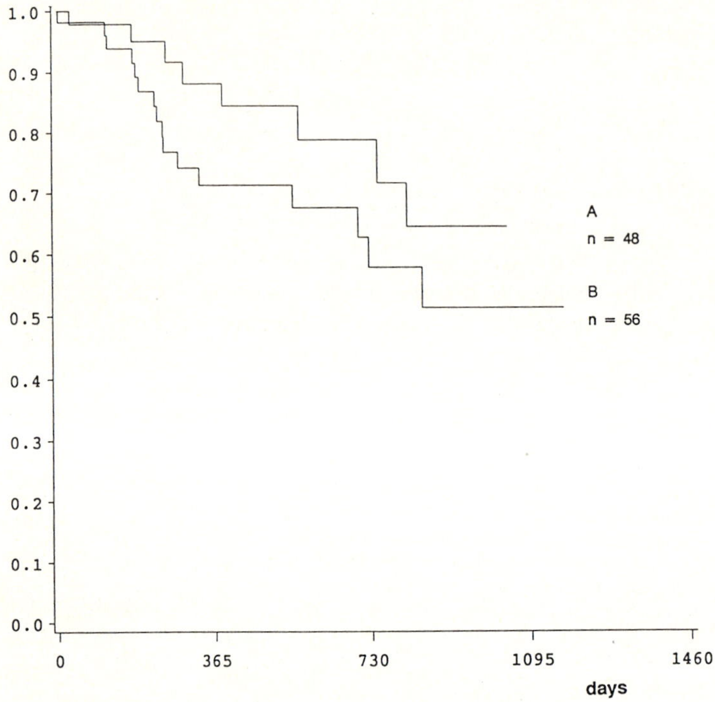

Fig. 1. German, Austrian, and Swiss Association for Head and Neck tumors study: Life table analysis in complete remission

in group A 85% male and 15% female and in group B 84% male and 16% female. The tumor localization is also similar in both groups, being mainly the floor of the mouth, tongue, lower and upper jaw, retromolar region, and the cheek.

So far in group A there are three local recurrences, two lymph node recurrences, two lymph node metastases, and two distant metastases. In group B there are nine local recurrences, four lymph node recurrences, two lymph node metastases, and no distant metastases. In group A, 37 out of 48 patients are still alive; the relative mortality is 23%. In group B, 43 out of 56 patients are still alive; again, the relative mortality is 23%. In Figs. 1 and 2, the life table analysis is shown for patients in primary complete remission and for patients still alive; there is no significant difference between the two treatment groups.

Discussion

Surgeons who support radical surgical treatment object to conservative neck dissection, arguing that lymph nodes containing metastases may be left. The

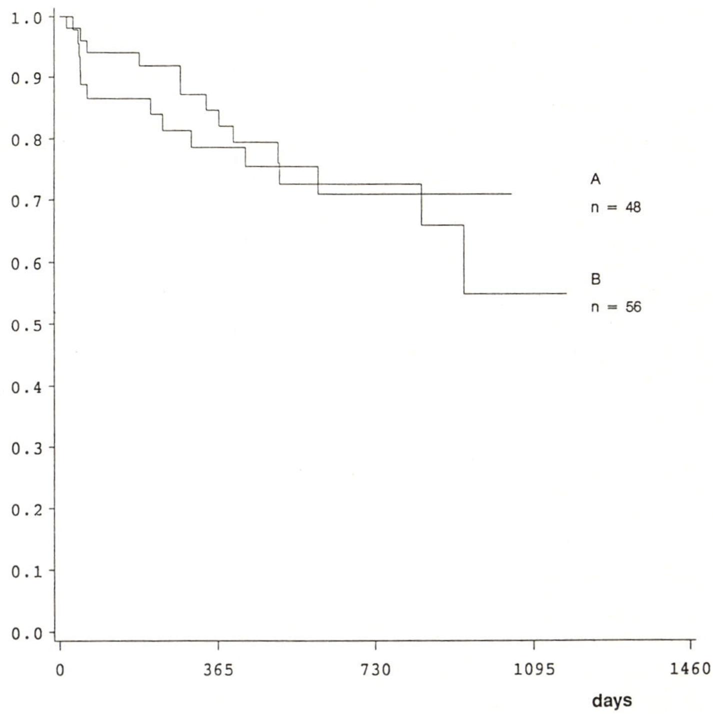

Fig. 2. German, Austrian, and Swiss Association for Head and Neck Tumors: Life table analysis for patients still alive

extent of this problem is particularly well illustrated by the discussion about the conservation of the accessory nerve.

As far as positive nodes at the accessory nerve in patients with oral squamous cell carcinomas are concerned, different results are reported in the literature. Among 225 patients with neck dissection, Skolnik et al. (1967) revealed positive accessory nerve nodes in 4% of the cases; unfortunately, these results were not differentiated according to negative and positive neck nodes. Results presented by Roy and Bears (1969) obtained in patients with clinically positive neck nodes histologically revealed only 0.4% positive nodes, a percentage ten times lower than the study presented by Skolnik et al. (1967).

Other authors have emphasized that in those cases with histologically positive nodes around the accessory nerve, multiple lymph node metastases in all other areas of the neck would also be present. It is remarkable that all these papers only address the lymph nodes at the accessory nerve, while other structures which are not removed during conservative neck dissection are not mentioned; this applies especially for the jugular vein, the platysma, and the sternoclei domastoid muscle.

Therefore, there is no real reason to argue against the preservation of structures during conservative neck dissection. However, as a result of ongoing DÖSAK study, we hope to clarify some questions regarding radical and conservative neck dissection.

Acknowledgements. The following clinical associates and clinics participated in this study: Auler, Mönchengladbach, Germany, Dieckmann, Recklinghausen, Germany, Ehrenfeld, Tübingen, Germany, Engleder, Linz, Austria, Gaebel, Karlsruhe, Germany, Grätz, Zürich, Switzerland, Honigmann, Basel, Switzerland, Howaldt, Frankfurt, Germany, Joenck, Kiel, Germany, Metelmann, Berlin-Steglitz, Germany, Mohr, Essen, Germany, Reuter, Bremerhaven, Germany, Risse, Aachen, Germany, Samek, Cologne, Germany, Scheibe, Augsburg, Germany, Schmelzeisen, Hanover University, Germany, Schmit, Henrietta-Stiftung, Hanover, Germany, Schwipper, Münster, Germany, Stoll, Freiburg, Germany, Toschka, Berlin-Virchow, Germany, Wagner, Mainz, Germany, Zahn, Bochum, Germany.

References

Ackermann K, Funk N, Fürg N (1985) Statistische Ergebnisse zur Therapie der Karzinome der Mundhöhle. Dtsch Z Mund Kiefer Gesichtschir 9:445–460

Bier J (1982) Definitionen zum radikalchirurgischen Vorgehen bei Plattenepithelkarzinomen der Mundhöhle. Dtsch Z Mund Kiefer Gesichtschir 6:369–372

Bocca E (1966) Supraglottic laryngectomy and functional neck dissection. J Laryngol Otol 80:831–838

Bocca E, Pignataro O (1967) A conservation technique in radical neck dissection. Ann Otol Rhinol Laryngol 76:975–987

Bocca E, Pignataro O, Oldini C, Cappa C (1984) Functional neck dissection: an evaluation and review of 843 cases. Laryngoscope 94:942–945

Byers RM (1985) Modified neck dissection. Am J Surg 150:414–421

Crile G (1906) Excision of cancer of the head and neck. JAMA 47:1780–1786

Kinsey DL, James AG (1962) The value of prophylactic neck dissection for cancer of the tongue. Surgery 51:155–160

Medina JE, Byers RM (1989) Supraomohyoid neck dissection: rationale, indications, and surgical technique. Head Neck 11:111–122

O'Brien CJ, Soong SJ, Urist M, Maddox WA (1987) Is modified radical neck dissection only a staying procedure? Cancer 59:994–999

O'Brien CJ, Urist MM, Maddox WA (1987b) Modified radical neck dissection: terminology, technique and indications. Am J Surg 153:310–316

Platz H, Hudec M (1986) Ergebnisse zur prospektiven und retrospektiven DÖSAK-Studie. DÖSAK-Arbeitstagung Hannover

Roy PH, Bears SOH (1969) Spinal accessory nerve in radical neck dissections. Am J Surg 118:800–804

Skolnik EM, Tenta LT, Wineinger DM, Tardy ME (1967) Preservation of XI cranial nerve in neck dissections. Laryngoscope 77:1304–1314

Southwick HW, Sloughter DP, Trevieso ET (1967) Elective neck dissection in intraoral cancer. Arch Surg 80:905–911

Suen JY, Goepfert H (1987) Standardization of neck dissection nomenclature (editorial). Head Neck Surg 10:75–77

Vandenbrouck C, Sancho-Garnier H, Chassagne D, Savarane D, Cachin Y, Micheau C (1980) Elective versus therapeutic radical neck dissection in epidermoid carcinoma of the oral cavity. Cancer 46:386–390

Treatment of Oropharynx Carcinomas: Experience at the Institut Gustave-Roussy

F. Eschwège[1], P. Wibault[1], A. Lusinchi[1], A. Gerbaulet[1], P. Marandas[2], C. Domenge[2], and B. Luboinski[2]

[1] Department of Radiotherapy, Institut Gustave-Roussy, rue Camille-Desmoulins, 94805 Villejuif, France
[2] Department of Head and Neck Surgery, Institut Gustave-Roussy, rue Camille-Desmoulins, 94805 Villejuif, France

Radiotherapy (RT) alone is the preferred treatment of oropharynx carcinomas T1, T2, N0, and N1 at the Institut Gustave-Roussy (IGR). More advanced or ulcerative tumors are treated with surgery combined with RT. For this type of tumor, induction chemotherapy (CT) before RT or surgery was recently used in our institute. Combined use of radiosensitizer and RT was also carried out recently in a European trial. For more advanced tumors, combined chemoradiotherapy and hyperfractionated schedule of RT were used in other phase II trials. Part of the experience with these forms of treatment is reported here.

Radiotherapy Alone in T1 and T2 Tumors in the Tonsillar Area

From 1970 to 1982, 193 T1 and T2 tumors have been treated with external RT alone; all of these were squamous cell carcinoma (SCC; 170 men, 23 women), 48 patients had T1 tumors, and 145 T2 tumors. Half of the patients (49%) presented with palpable nodes, and 82 out of 96 had ipsilateral subdigastric nodes. Patients were treated with cobalt 60 with a minimum dose of 50 Gy over 5 weeks (4–5 fractions a week) for the primary and cervical area. A boost of the primary area of 20–25 Gy was given (mean total dose, 71.6 Gy). The dose applied to uninvolved nodes was 50 Gy, and 65 Gy over 6.5 weeks to the palpable nodes.

Immediate results were excellent: 86% of tumor patients had complete remission (CR). The percentage of patients with CR was higher for T1 (96%) and superficial tumors (93%) than for T2 (83%) and nodular (more than 5 mm thick) tumors (83%). Two months after the end of RT, there was residual disease only in four patients, and nodal response in 89 of 95 patients (94%). As far as local control was concerned, 34 local recurrences were observed (total failures, 9.6%). In 58% of these the local recurrence occurred at the margin of the treated volume, particularly in the case of superficial tumors (86%); 21 of 34 could be successfully salvaged; 14 of the 21 (67%) were salvaged by means of transmaxillary buccopharyngectomy. Local control 2 years after the end of RT was 81% for the whole group, 88% for the T1 group, 79% for the T2 group (not significant, NS), 75% for superficial tumors, and 83% for nodular ones. Local spread was a prognostic factor for local control: in ten of 30 patients with tumors extending forwards to the anterior pillar, recurrences were observed. Ninety-four percent of N0 tumors, 92% of N1 tumors, 100% of N2 tumors, and only 59% of N3 tumors were controlled. Nineteen patients (10%) had metastases: 5 years after the end of RT, 39% of N3 patients had metastases, compared to 5% in the other groups.

The most important complication was osteonecrosis (28 patients); a hemimandibulectomy was performed in 11 patients. Most cases of osteonecrosis occurred at sites of dental extraction prior to treatment. The survival rate was 73% at 3 years and 58% at 5 years, and survival was not related either to stage (T1, 64%; T2, 56%) or to the macroscopic appearance, but it was related to the nodal status (62.5% for N0, 64% for N1 and N2, but only 34.5% for N3 patients). The 5-year survival rate was 70% for poorly differentiated tumors versus 55% for well-differentiated ones (p, 0.005; Lusinchi et al. 1989).

Base of Tongue Carcinoma

The treatment of this tumor is external RT alone or combined external RT and brachytherapy for T1, T2, and some T3 tumors. This treatment was undertaken from 1961 to 1983 in 108 patients (18 T1 tumors, 39 T2 tumors, and 51 T3 tumors). The mean dose of external RT was 46 Gy (30–70 Gy); following this treatment, complete response was obtained in 61% of T1 patients, 28% of T2 patients, and 14% of T3 patients. Brachytherapy was done using either a guide gutter or plastic tubes, with a mean dose of 43.8 Gy (22–84 Gy); the mean cumulative dose was 89 Gy (67–142 Gy). Local control at 5 years was obtained in 64% (37 failures out of 108), with 58% in T1 patients, 50% in T2 patients, and 69% in T3 patients; 29 cases of necrosis were observed (27%). Nodal control was observed in 82% for N0 and 79% in palpable nodes. The 5-year survival rate was 26%: 53% for T1 patients, 16% for T2 patients, and 24% for T3 patients, with a significant number of second cancer and metastases in patients who consumed considerable amounts of alcohol and/or were heavy smokers (Lusinchi et al. 1989).

In oropharynx tumors, for limited tumors (T1 and T2) and for some selected locations, external RT alone, or combined with brachytherapy, is able to control primary tumors and nodes; the 5-year survival rate is often poor due to the impact of metastases and second primary tumors.

Beside the surgical possibilities (transmandibular pharyngectomy) and postoperative radiotherapy, the following questions have been discussed: (a) is the use of radiosensitizer combined with RT superior to RT alone? and (b) is induction CT able to improve local control and survival?

Radiosensitizer Trial

A European randomized trial has been done to compare radiotherapy alone (70 Gy five times per week) to RT and 2 g etanidazole (SR 2508)/m^2 three times per week (a total of 34 g/m^2 in 17 infusions). Oropharynx carcinomas at the T2, T3, or T4 and N0, N1, or N2 stage with a hemoglobin level of more than 11 g/l. were irradiated, as were supraglottic, glottic larynx, and hypopharynx carcinoma. The first results have no shown major toxicities, and there was no difference in the cumulative regression rate between the two groups; neither local control and survival data nor data concerning the development of the oropharynx subgroup itself are yet available.

Induction Chemotherapy

From 1986 to 1991, The French Groupe de Traitement des Tumeurs de la Tête et du Cou (GETTEC) carried out a randomized trial (chimiothérapie des cancers de l'oropharynx, CHIMORO) to compare induction CT followed by external RT with RT alone. The Al Sarraf schedule was chosen (fluorouracil, 5-Fu, and cisplatyl, CDDP). A total of 174 patients with SCC of the oropharynx (vallecula and posterior pharyngeal wall excluded) at the T2, T3, or T4 and N0, N1, or N2a,b,c, less than 70 years of age, WHO grades I and II, were randomized (86 in CT-RT arm and 88 in RT arm). In the CT arm, complete or partial remission was achieved in 67.5% of the patients; with the same follow-up time, no differences have been seen in terms of recurrence rate and survival between the two groups (Table 1).

Table 1. Follow-up results of the CHIMORO study

	CT and RT (n = 86)	RT (n = 88)
Alive	56 (65%)	47 (53%) NS
Disease-free	43 (77%)	39 (83%) NS
Second cancer	1	3
Intercurrent	7	1
Posttreatment	1	–

CT, induction chemotherapy; RT, radiotherapy, NS, not significant.

A trial comparing induction CT before surgery and postoperative RT with surgery and postop erative RT with the same CT regimen was undertaken by GETTEC during the same period. The first analyses have shown no differences in terms of local control and survival.

For more advanced tumors, the treatment of choice is surgery with postoperative RT. For very advanced tumors, results of surgery and postoperative RT and conventional RT are poor. In some cases, a curative surgical approach is impossible, due to significant local or nodal extension. Combined radiochemotherapy or accelerated, hyperfractionated RT techniques are used in our department in phase II trials.

Combined Radiochemotherapy

This schedule of treatment is not strictly limited to oropharynx cancer; it is used in our department for patients with advanced head and neck tumors which cannot be cured by RT treatment alone in normal fractionation or by surgery and which are not suitable for hyperfractionated treatment (see below).

From 1987 to 1990, 29 patients with SCC (oropharynx, 13; larynx, 3; hypopharynx, 7; others, 6) – all T4 and/or N3 M0 – were treated with combined RT (70 Gy over 7 weeks), cisplatin 80 mg/m^2 IV on days 5, 27, and 49, and 5-FU in continuous infusion (300 mg 7 weeks). Three months after completion of RT, complete remission was achieved in 46% of the patients, 66% for tT, 52% for N. Local control (no evidence of disease, NED, >3 months) was obtained in nine out of 28 patients, with an average follow-up of 12 months (4+, 35+). Thirteen patients are alive, 8 NED. All patients have had enteral nutrition; mucositis grade 3/4 (WHO/Radiation Therapy Oncology Group (RTOG) criteria) was found in 83% of the patients. One patient died early, and one renal toxicity (CDDP related) was observed. This regimen is feasible with good local control and the possibility of curative results, but we do not know whether it is superior to RT alone.

Hyperfractionated and Accelerated Irradiation

For very advanced tumors with nonposterior nodal extension not suitable for curative surgery or RT, a course of accelerated irradiation was chosen (Lusinchi et al. 1991). A total of 47 patients were treated from 1988 to 1990 (40 T4 and 42 N0 or N1). The total dose was 70 Gy to the primary area over 5.5 weeks (three fractions of 0.9 Gy a day, with 4 h intervals; spinal cord reduction at 37.8 Gy, inferior cervical nodes receiving 50 Gy in 25 fractions). Tolerance was fair, but nasogastric feeding was necessary in 20 patients;

grade 3 mucositis was found in 26 patients, but moist skin desquamation in only one, and only one patient had a soft tissue necrosis.

Three months after irradiation, complete tumor response was obtained in 79% of patients (37 out of 47), and complete nodal response in 18 out of 18 patients. At 2 years, local control was obtained in 41% of the patients; the 2-year survival was 26.4%, which is high for patients with a very considerable extension (total tongue extension in 11 cases, soft tissue involvement in 15 cases, bone involvement in six cases, and tumoral trismus in eight cases).

In order to achieve the correct tolerance, two new accelerated irradiation schedules are in progress in our department. In the first protocol for T3, T4, N0, and N1 tumors, the total dose is 70 Gy delivered over 27 days in 3 fractions (0.9, 0.9, and 1.4 Gy) at 4-h intervals. Another, more accelerated protocol is designed for patients with N2 or N3 nodes, with 62 Gy over 19 days (2 fractions of 1.75 Gy at 10-h intervals) with irradiation on the Saturday (i.e. day 6).

Work in Progress

Choosing treatment in oropharynx carcinoma is not easy. A biological approach may be used to facilitate this choice. Knowledge of some factors may be useful before treatment (Cosset et al. 1990):

1. Knowledge of the oxygenation of tumors is now possible by use of polarographic evaluation (measurement of PaO_2 inside tumor, nodes, or normal tissue; Lartigau 1992).
2. Appreciation of the speed of tumor development, measuring the potential doubling time (T_{pot}), and/or labeling index. This T_{pot} seems to be a very important prognostic factor that can be obtained by biopsy. It allows an appreciation of the rapidity of the tumor development and the possible suitability of the accelerated irradiation schedule (Bourhis et al. 1991).

Conclusion

The evolution of the treatment of oropharynx tumors at the IGR reflects the modification of ideas over the past 20 years. The choice of treatment in each individual case is based on the site of the tumor, presence or absence of nodes, the Karnofsky index, and macro- and microscopic aspects, but may also be based on the biological characteristics of the tumor. The fact that the 5- and 10-year survival rates are no different than those recorded 5 or 10 years ago may be due to the impact of second cancers.

References

Bourhis J, Wilson GD, Janot F, Chavaudra N, Leridant AM, Wibault P, Girinsky T, Luboinski B, Eschwege F, Malaise EP (1991) Mesure de la cinétique de prolifération in vivo des cancers de l'oropharynx par incorporation de bromodésoxyruridine et cytométrie de flux. Bull Cancer 78:1045–1051

Cosset JL, Peters LJ, Girinsky T, Guichard M, Eschwege F, Mornex F, Malaise EP (1990) Les tests prédictifs de radiosensibilité. Vers une radiothérapie sur mesure. Bull Cancer Radiother 77:83–84

Lartigau E (1992) Oxygenation of head and neck tumors. Radiation Research Society, 40th annual meeting, workshop geographic physiology of tumors. Salt Lake City

Lusinchi A, Eskandari J, Son Y, Gerbaulet A, Haie C, Mamelle G, Eschwege F, Chassagne D (1989a) External irradiation plus curietherapy boost in 108 base of tongue carcinoma. Int J Radiat Oncol Biol Phys 99:1257–1259

Lusinchi A, Wibault P, Marandas P, Kunkler I, Eschwege F (1989) Exclusive radiation therapy: the treatment of early tonsillar tumors. Int J Radiat Oncol Biol Phys 17:273–277

Lusinchi A, Wibault P, Luboinski B, Eschwege F (1991) Accelerated radiation therapy. The treatment of very advanced head and neck carcinoma. ECCO 6, Florence Oct 1991, Eur J Cancer 27 [Suppl]:2, Abstract 829

Concomitant Boost-Accelerated, Superfractionated Irradiation for the Treatment of Advanced Carcinomas of the Oral Cavity and Oropharynx

R.K. Schmidt-Ullrich[1], C.R. Johnson[1], S. Khandelwal[1], and D.E. Wazer[2]

[1] Department of Radiation Oncology, Medical College of Virginia, Richmond, VA, USA
[2] Department of Radiation Oncology, Tufts-New England Medical Center, Boston, MA, USA

Introduction

With the trend of organ-preserving cancer management, the treatment of squamous cell carcinomas (SCC) of the upper aerodigestive tract increasingly includes radiotherapy used alone or in combination with surgery. The current standards of maximum locoregional tumor control of more advanced SCC of the oral cavity and oropharynx have been set by surgical resection combined with pre- or postoperative irradiation yielding widely varying control rates depending on tumor site and stage (Wazer et al. 1989; Huang et al. 1992; Parsons et al. 1981; Chu and Fletcher 1973; Million 1979; Dasmahapatra et al. 1986). Similar control rates have been achieved for moderately advanced lesions of the oral cavity using combined external beam and interstitial irradiation (Schmidt-Ullrich et al. 1991a; Mendenhall et al. 1981; Fu et al. 1976; Wang et al. 1983). Based on recent investigation, superfractionated and accelerated irradiation has been applied to the treatment of carcinomas of the oral cavity and oropharynx (Peters et al. 1988; Withers et al. 1988; Wang 1988; Saunders et al. 1989; Million et al. 1985; Horiot et al. 1988; Schmidt-Ullrich et al. 1991b; Ang et al. 1990; Johnson et al. 1992).

In our prospective, nonrandomized study at the Tufts-New England Medical (T-NEMC) and the Medical College of Virginia (MCV), we have irradiated patients with advanced carcinomas of the upper aerodigestive tract with twice daily (b.i.d.) radiotherapy using the concomitant boost technique, which delivers the second daily treatment to a reduced volume (Schmidt-Ullrich et al. 1991; Ang et al. 1990; Johnson et al. 1992). Comparison to once daily (qd) radiotherapy at the same institutions, T-NEMCH and MCV, revealed that patients with advanced head and neck malignancies treated with b.i.d. irradiation experienced significantly improved tumor control, disease-free, and overall survival rates (Wang 1988; Sanders 1989; Million et al. 1985; Horiot et al. 1988; Schmidt-Ullrich et al. 1991b; Ang et al. 1990; Parsons et al. 1988). We report here that these findings also apply to a subgroup of 75 patients irradiated for American Joint Commission on Cancer (AJCC) stage III and IV SCC of the oral cavity/oropharynx. Computed tomography (CT)-based volume analyses of tumor sizes has resulted in the definition of tumor volumes that have a high likelihood of being controlled with b.i.d. radiotherapy alone.

Material and Methods

Patients

Of the patients with SCC of the oral cavity and oropharynx irradiated with curative intent at T-NEMC and MCV, 34 patients were treated qd and 41 were irradiated b.i.d. In both institutions, the patients treated b.i.d. since 1985 and 1988 at T-NEMC and MCV, respectively, were compared to patients irradiated qd in the immediately preceding years. The minimum follow-up of all patients is 12 months after diagnosis with an actuarial follow-up projected to 50 months. The male to female ratios in the qd and b.i.d. groups were 26:8 and 34:7, respectively.

The patients were staged according to the AJCC staging system (American Joint Commission on Cancer 1988) with T- and N-stage distributions as specified in Table 1. The staging work-up included physical examination, CT scans of the head and neck region and the chest, panendoscopy, and routine blood chemistries. Eligible were patients with Karnovsky performance scales of 70% or better.

Table 1. T and N stages of patients with advanced squamous cell carcinoma of the oral cavity and oropharynx

	T1	T2	T3	T4	Total
Once daily					
N0	0	0	1	0	1
N1	0	6	0	2	8
N2	6	2	4	3	15
N3	4	1	3	2	10
Total	10	9	8	7	34
Twice daily					
N0	0	0	0	0	0
N1	1	2	5	0	8
N2	8	2	3	0	13
N3	6	3	4	7	20
Total	15	7	12	7	41

Estimation of Tumor Volumes

The volumes of primary tumors were computed from diagnostic CT scans obtained after intravenous contrast administration. The CT scans were viewed over a light box and digitized with a DAGE-MTI 81 video camera and software/hardware including a Compaq 386/25 computer (Loats Associates, Winchester, MD). After video image capture, tumor areas were outlined using a Micro Digi-pad (GTCO, Columbia, MD) and the total delineated area was calculated by the computer. The tumor volumes of each CT slice were obtained from the tumor area and the slice thickness. The total tumor volumes were computed by summation of all tumor slice volumes. For some of the very large tumors, extension into the soft tissues of the neck was judged as primary tumor. This may have resulted in overestimation of the size of some very large primary tumors which tend to be contiguous with lymph node metastases.

Radiotherapy Schedules

Details of the radiotherapy schedules have been published elsewhere (Schmidt-Ullrich et al. 1991; Johnson et al. 1992; Table 2). Shortly, patients irradiated qd were treated with 1.8 Gy fractions to the tumor and the lymph node areas of the neck and supraclavicular region at risk to a dose of 50.4 Gy followed by boosts to clinical disease to total doses of 68.4–72.0 Gy. The duration of this treatment course was about 54 days. The group of patients treated b.i.d. was irradiated with the same continuous course as the qd cohort, delivering 50.4 Gy to the entire head and neck region. Except for seven patients, all received the concomitant boost irradiation to clinical disease between days 22 and 42 (Table 2). The second 1.6-Gy fraction was given with a minimum interval of 4 h thrice a week on Monday, Wednesday,

Table 2. Accelerated superfractionation and standard fractionation for advanced squamous cell carcinoma of upper aerodigestive tract

Weeks	Dose
B.i.d. schedule	
1–3	1.8 Gy × 13
4–6	1.8 Gy × 15 + 1.6 Gy × 9 (reduced field)
7	1.8 Gy × 3 (reduced field)
Total	70.2 Gy
Qd schedule	
1–6	1.8 Gy × 28
7–8	1.8 Gy × 11 (reduced field)
Total	70.2 Gy

and Friday. The final boost to total doses of 68.4 Gy and 73.8 Gy was through further reduced portals. The duration of the b.i.d. schedule was about 45 days.

Radiotherapy Techniques

All patients were treated with megavoltage irradiation using ^{60}CO/80 units and 4/100 or 6/100 Varian linear accelerators. All patients treated on the b.i.d. protocol and most patients treated qd were irradiated through wedged lateral portals after CT-based treatment planning and a supraclavicular field. Doses were prescribed at the tumor level. The maximum accepted dose to the cervical spinal cord was 45 Gy. The cord was excluded from the second daily treatment of the b.i.d. schedule in all cases. The posterior neck nodes were irradiated through portals using 9 MeV electrons.

Assessment of Treatment Toxicity

Mucosal reactions and patient weights were recorded weekly as described before (Schmidt-Ullrich et al. 1991; Johnson et al. 1992). All patients were counselled to assure adequate nutritional intake and maintained on systemic ketoconazole to prevent deep mucosal *Candida* infections (Schmidt-Ullrich et al. 1991b).

Follow-up and Statistical Evaluations

Within the first and second year after completion of treatment, the patients were clinically evaluated monthly or bimonthly, respectively. In addition, the tumor status was evaluated with CT scans at 6-month intervals for the first 3 years and compared to a baseline study obtained 3 months after completion of treatment. Chest X-rays were obtained at 6-month intervals.

Actuarial local control and adjusted and overall survival rates were determined using the Kaplan-Meier method (Kaplan and Meier 1958).

Results

Patient Population

Only patients with a minimum of 12 months follow-up after diagnosis are included in the present analysis. The median follow-up times for the qd and b.i.d. groups are 19 months (range, 6–114 months) and 18 months (range, 5–80 months), respectively. Patients at risk in the qd and b.i.d. group are

Table 3. Distribution of squamous cell carcinoma in the qd and b.i.d. group by location of the primary sites

Site	Qd	B.i.d.
Floor of mouth	2	3
Oral tongue	0	2
Retromolar tongue	4	3
Tongue base	11	15
Tonsil area	7	9
Soft palate	1	4
Pharyngeal wall	9	5
Total	34	41

qd, *quaque die* (once daily); b.i.d., *bis in die* (twice daily)

three and 13, respectively. The distribution by T- and N-stages of the two treatment groups, as listed in Table 1, demonstrates a similar distribution in the qd and b.i.d. groups.

The distribution of primary tumors by site is given in Table 3. Except for the preponderance of pharyngeal wall carcinomas in the qd group, there is a similar representation of all tumors in both study groups.

Tumor Control and Patient Survival

The actuarial 50-month locoregional control rate of 62% for the b.i.d. group is significantly higher than the 17% rate for the qd group (p, 0.008; Fig. 1). With the exception of four patients, the local control rates are reported for radiotherapy alone. Only one patient in the b.i.d. group with an extensive T4 carcinoma of the anterior floor of mouth was resected 3 months after completion of radiotherapy and was found to have no residual viable tumor. Three patients in the qd group had salvage surgery within 3 months of irradiation. The improved tumor control rates translated into statistically significant adjusted and overall survival advantages at 50 months with p values of 0.006 and 0.03, respectively (Figs. 2, 3).

Tumor Volumes and Tumor Control

The volumes of primary tumors in the b.i.d. group demonstrated that for T2 and T3 lesions, the T-stage correlated well with volumes computed (Fig. 4). The relative lack of correlation for T4 carcinomas is due to the fact that small tumors are categorized as T4 lesions because of bone invasion and that massive tumors are frequently contiguous with lymph node disease in the neck. The volume ranges for T2, T3, and T4 tumors were 2–14 cm^3, 6–

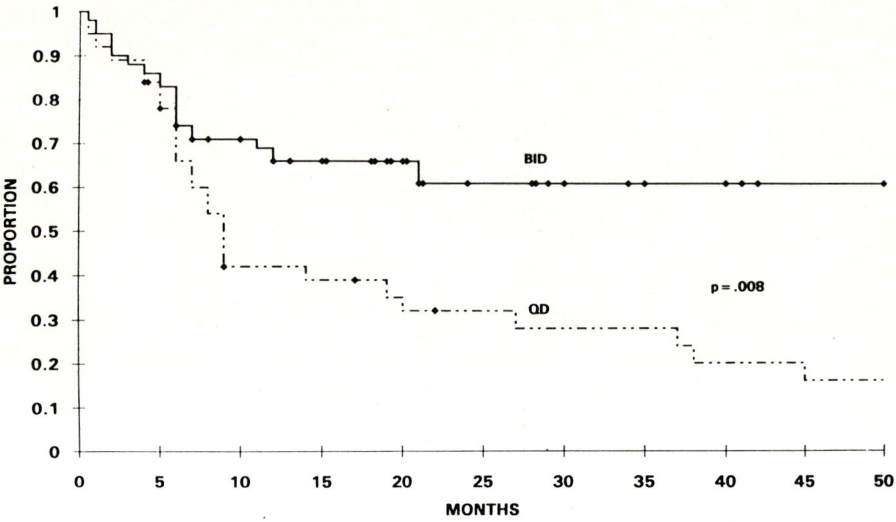

Fig. 1. Locoregional tumor control rates of patients treated with a qd and b.i.d. radiotherapy course

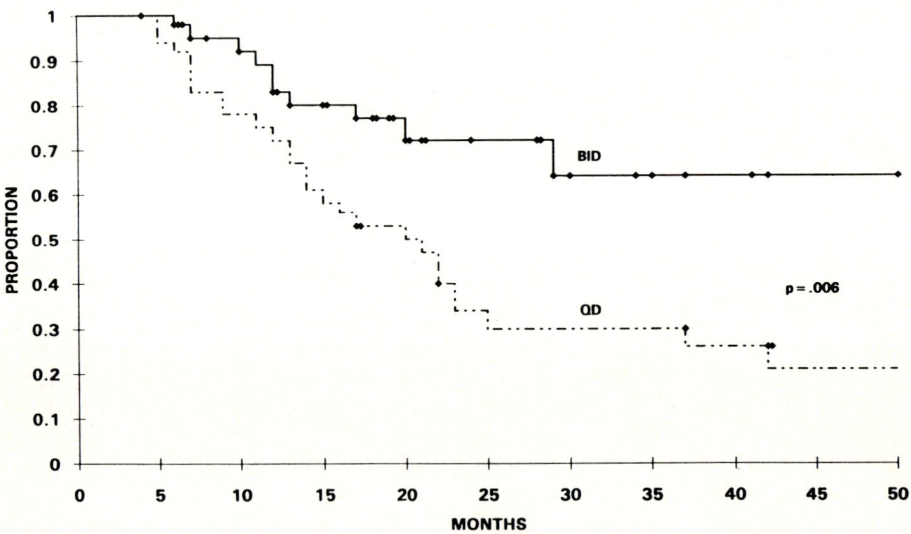

Fig. 2. Adjusted survival of patients treated with a qd and b.i.d. course of radiotherapy

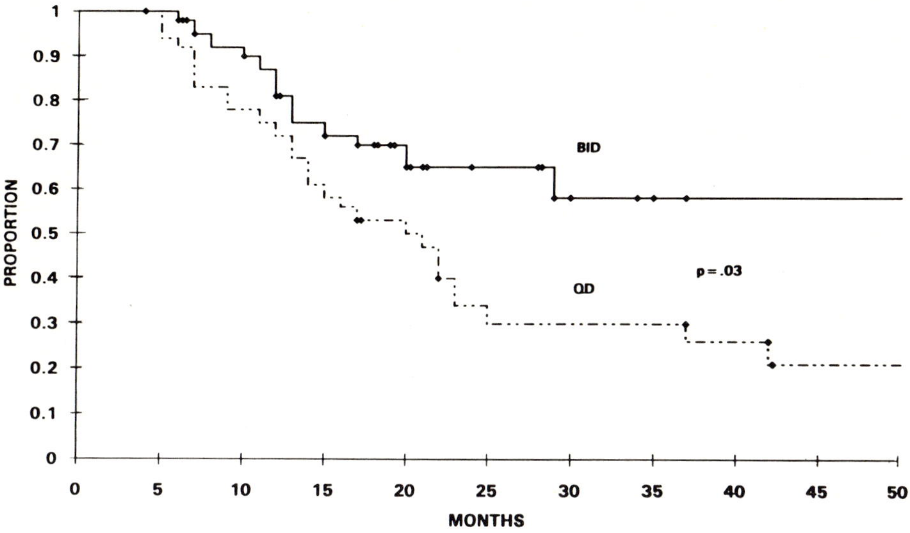

Fig. 3. Overall survival rates of patients treated with a qd and b.i.d. radiotherapy course

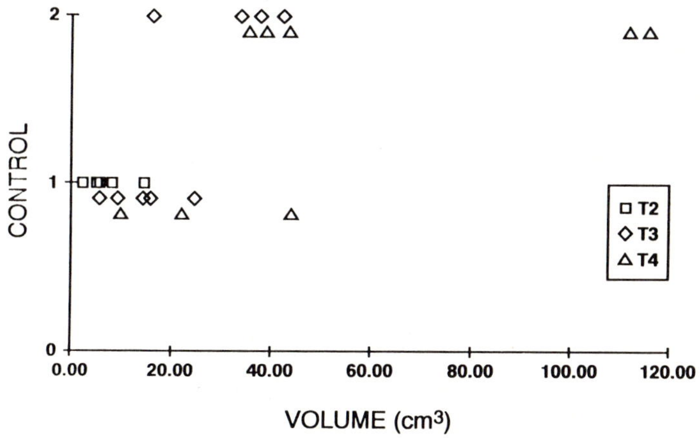

Fig. 4. Tumor control by T stage and tumor volume. The ordinate value gives tumor control: 1, controlled; 2, failure. The abscissa value gives tumor volume

42 cm^3, and 8–195 cm^3, respectively. With respect to tumor control, no failures were observed of tumors smaller than 15 cm^3. Tumors up to 42 cm^3 were controlled with radiotherapy alone. For tumors larger than 100 cm^3, it was impossible to separate primary carcinoma from contiguous nodal disease.

Tolerance and Response to Radiotherapy

Failures occurred at a similar rate in both treatment groups during the first 12 months, at which time the curves start to separate (Figs. 1–3). Patients failing after irradiation for massive tumors within 6 months most likely have persistent disease. This has been suggested by our previous finding that patients with complete tumor responses 3 months after completion of irradiation had superior lasting control rates (Johnson et al. 1992).

Complications

The acute and late complications in patients with SCC of oral cavity/oropharynx were similar to those of the entire study group (Schmidt-Ullrich et al. 1991; Johnson et al. 1992). Shortly, all patients in the b.i.d. group had grade 1, about 90% grade 2, about 50% grade 3, and 0% grade 4 mucosal reactions (van den Bogaert et al. 1986). While the acute toxicity of the b.i.d. schedule was greater, no treatment breaks were required. There has been no increase in late complications (Schmidt-Ullrich et al. 1991b; Johnson et al. 1992).

Discussion

The regimen of accelerated, superfractionated irradiation used for treatment of advanced SCC of the oral cavity and oropharynx has produced superior results with respect to locoregional tumor control and adjusted and overall survival at 50 months relative to the conventional qd regimen. Our results confirm those of other trials of superfractionation and accelerated superfractionation, which show similar improvements in locoregional tumor control, as long as the radiation dose is delivered over a relatively short time period (Fowler 1989; Johnson et al. 1992; Withers et al. 1988).

The schedule favoring superfractionation (Horiot et al. 1988; Million et al. 1985; Parsons et al. 1988) by delivering 1.2 Gy b.i.d. throughout the treatment course has been tested in institutional and randomized trials and was found to be superior to conventional schedules only if total radiation doses were escalated to 72–76 Gy (Parsons et al. 1988; Marcial et al. 1987).

The most challenging problem in the use of accelerated superfractionation is the avoidance of acute toxcity, which may interfere with the delivery of a continuous treatment course. This problem has been addressed in two ways. A regimen using relatively high fractions of 1.6 Gy b.i.d. to the entire head and neck region requires a treatment break of 11 days after day 16 of the treatment regimen (Wang 1988). After the break, patients can resume b.i.d. irradiation and complete the radiotherapy course in a significantly shorter time period (Fowler 1989; Wang 1988; Withers et al. 1988). The disadvantage of this regimen is that there is a potential for tumor repopulation during the 11-day break, which could counteract the effectiveness of treatment. Another regimen of extreme accelerated superfractionation delivers 1.5 Gy thrice daily to a total dose of 54 Gy in 12 consecutive days (Saunders et al. 1989). The most severe toxicity of this regimen does not manifest itself until the course is completed. Patients are managed for their complications during the 2 months following radiotherapy. The regimen of concomitant boost-accelerated superfractionation, explored at two institutions (Schmidt-Ullrich et al. 1991b; Ang et al. 1990), delivers the same nominal dose of about 70 Gy during 45 instead of 54 days and uses b.i.d. irradiation during the second part of the treatment course when repopulation is thought to be most dominant (Withers et al. 1988; Fowler 1989). For further improved tolerance, reduced portals were used for the b.i.d. phase of the treatment course. This schedule has allowed the delivery of high-dose irradiation with a shortening of the continuous course by about 10 days and has resulted in significantly improved tumor control and survival rates (Schmidt-Ullrich et al. 1991b; Johnson et al. 1992).

Tumor volume analyses using modern imaging and volume reconstruction techniques are evolving as important tools for the prediction of treatment outcome and determination of the need of combined modality versus single modality treatment. The analysis of 21 tumors in the b.i.d. group showed that tumors of up to 43 cm^3 were controlled using our accelerated superfractionation schedule and that no failures were seen with tumors of 15 cm^3 or less. While we could not obtain original high-quality CT scans of patients treated qd, similar analyses on patients irradiated for laryngeal carcinomas according to standard schedules exist and have demonstrated that tumors with volumes of about 9 cm^3 or less have a high likelihood of being controlled by radiotherapy alone (Freeman et al. 1990; Gilbert et al. 1987).

In summary, the accelerated superfractionation schedule used in this study results in superior tumor control and survival of patients with advanced SCC of the upper aerodigestive tract. While patients irradiated b.i.d. experience a somewhat increased acute toxicity, this does not preclude delivery of a continuous treatment course and does not translate into increased late complications. Our schedule of concomitant b.i.d. irradiation using a continuous course of standard radiotherapy supplemented with reduced field boosts during weeks 4 to 6 allows shortening of the overall treatment time by 10 days. The regimen allows for further reduction of the treatment time by integration of a thrice-daily scheduling into a standard continuous radiotherapy course. Such a pilot study is being conducted at our institution.

References

American Joint Commission on Cancer (1988) Manual for staging of cancer. Lippincott, Philadelphia

Ang KK, Peters LJ, Weber RS, Maor MH, Morrison WH, Wendt CD (1990) Concomitant boost radiotherapy schedules in the treatment of carcinoma of the oropharynx and nasopharynx. Int J Radiat Oncol Biol Phys 19:1339–1345

Chu A, Fletcher GH (1973) Incidence and causes of failures to control by irradiation the primary tumors in squamous cell carcinoma of the anterior two-thirds of the tongue and floor of mouth. Am J Roentgenol 117:502–508

Dasmahapatra K, Mirseyed A, Rush B, Hill G, Feurerman M, Ohanian M (1986) Cancer of the tonsil – improved survival with combination therapy. Cancer 57: 451–455

Fowler JF (1989) The linear-quadratic formula and progress in fractionated radiotherapy. Br J Radiol 62:679–694

Freeman DE, Mancuso AA, Parsons JT, Mendenhall WM, Million RR (1990) Irradiation alone for supraglottic larynx carcinoma: can CT findings predict treatment results? Int J Radiat Oncol Biol Phys 19:485–490

Fu KK, Ray JY, Chang EK, Phillips TL (1976) External and interstitial radiationtherapy of carcinoma of oral tongue. Am J Roentgenol 126:107–115

Gilbert RW, Birt D, Shulman H, Freeman J et al. (1987) Correlation of tumor volume with local control in laryngeal carcinoma treated by radiotherapy. Ann Otol Rhinol Laryngol 96:514–518

Horiot JC, Le Fur R, Nguyen T et al. (1988) Two fractions per day versus a single fraction per day in the radiotherapy of oropharynx carcinoma: results of an EORTC randomized trial. Proceedings of the 30th annual ASTRO meeting 123:179

Huang D, Johnson CR, Schmidt-Ullrich RK, Sismanis A, Neifeld JP, Weber J (1992) Incompletely resected advanced squamous cell carcinoma of the head and neck: the effectiveness of adjuvant vs. salvage radiotherapy. Radiother Oncol 23 (in press)

Johnson CR, Schmidt-Ullrich RK, Wazer DE (1992) Concomitant boost technique using accelerated superfractionated radiation therapy for advanced squamous cell carcinoma of the head and neck. Cancer 69:2749–2754

Kaplan EL, Meier P (1958) Nonparametric estimation from incomplete observations. J Am Stat Assoc 53:457–481

Marcial VA, Pajak TF, Chang C, Tupchong L, Stetz J (1987) Hyperfractionated photon radiation therapy in the treatment of advanced squamous cell carcinoma of the oral cavity, pharynx, larynx, and sinuses, using radiation therapy as the only planned modality (preliminary report). Int J Radiat Oncol Biol Phys 13:41–47

Mendenhall WM, Steed Van Cise W, Bova FJ, Million RR (1981) Analysis of time–dose factors in squamous cell carcinomas of the oral tongue and floor of mouth treated with radiation therapy alone. Int J Radiat Oncol Biol Phys 7: 1005–1011

Million RR (1979) Squamous cell carcinoma of the head and neck: combined therapy: surgery and postoperative irradiation. Int J Radiat Oncol Biol Phys 5:2161–2162

Million RR, Parsons JT, Cassisi NJ (1985) Twice-a-day irradiation technique for squamous cell carcinomas of the head and neck. Cancer 55:2096–2099

Parsons JT, Million RR, Cassisi NJ (1981) Carcinoma of the base of the tongue: results of radical irradiation with surgery reserved for irradiation failure. Laryngoscope 92:689–696

Parsons JT, Mendenhall WM, Cassisi NJ, Isaacs JH Jr, Million RR (1988) Hyperfractionation for head and neck cancer. Int J Radiat Oncol Biol Phys 14:649–658

Peters LJ, Ang KK, Thomas HD (1988) Accelerated fractionation the radiation treatment of head and neck cancer: a critical comparison of different treatment strategies. Acta Oncol 27 [Suppl 2]:185–194

Saunders MI, Dische S, Hong A et al. (1989) Continuous hyperfractionated accelerated radiotherapy in locally advanced carcinoma of the head and neck region. Int J Radiat Oncol Biol Phys 17:1287–1293

Schmidt-Ullrich RK, Zwicker RD, Wu A, Kelly A (1991a) Interstitial IR-192 implants of the oral cavity: the planning and construction of volume implants. Int J Radiat Oncol Biol Phys 20:1079–1085

Schmidt-Ullrich RK, Johnson CR, Wazer DE, Masko G, Chasin WD, Karmody CS (1991b) Accelerated superfractionated irradiation for advanced carcinoma of the head and neck: concomitant boost technique. Int J Radiat Oncol Biol Phys 21:563–568

van den Bogaert W, Van der Schueren E, Horiot J-C et al. (1986) Early results of the EORTC randomized clinical trial on multiple fractions per day (MFD) and misonidazole in advanced head and neck cancer. Int J Radiat Oncol Biol Phys 12:587–591

Wang CC (1988) Local control of oropharyngeal carcinoma after two accelerated hyperfractionation radiation therapy schemes. Int J Radiat Oncol Biol Phys 14: 1143–1146

Wang CC, Doppke KP, Bridges PJ (1983) Intraoral cone radiation therapy for selected carcinomas of the oral cavity. Int J Radiat Oncol Biol Phys 9:1185–1189

Wazer DE, Schmidt-Ullrich RK, Keisch M, Karmody CS, Koch W (1989) The role of combined composite resection and irradiation in the management of carcinoma of the oral cavity and oropharynx. Strahlenther Onkol 165:18–22

Withers HR, Taylor JMG, Maciejewski B (1988) The hazard of accelerated tumor clonogen repopulation during radiotherapy. Acta Oncol 27 [Suppl 2]:131–146

Regional Lymph Node Irradiation

J.T. Parsons, R.R. Million, and W.M. Mendenhall

Department of Radiation Oncology, University of Florida Health Science Center, P.O. Box 100385, Gainesville, FL 32610-0385, USA

Management of the Clinically Negative Neck

When the lymph ondes are clinically negative (N0) and the risk of subclinical disease is 10%–15% or greater, the lymph nodes are included in the treatment portals and receive a minimum dose equivalent to 4500 cGy over 4½ weeks. In some clinical situations, the first-echelon nodes receive a much higher dose incidental to irradiation of the primary lesion. In the treatment portals used for cancers of the oropharynx, larynx, and hypopharynx, most of the high-risk neck nodes are encompassed by slight enlargement of the portals used to include the primary lesion. The decision to use elective lymph node irradiation depends on several factors:

1. Primary site and its relative density of capillary lymphatics
2. Risk of bilateral subclinical disease
3. Histologic grade and vascular space invasion
4. Depth of invasion and size of the primary lesion
5. Difficulty of neck examination
6. Relative morbidity for extending the lymph node coverage related to the risk of subclinical disease
7. Likelihood that the patient will return for frequent follow-up examinations
8. Suitability of the patient for a radical neck dissection should tumor appear in the neck

A policy of "wait and see" may be adopted for the N0 neck in patients who are at low risk of lymph node metastasis (e.g., T1–T2 N0 true vocal cord cancer, T1 N0 well-differentiated floor of mouth cancer, nasal vestibule cancer, etc.) in order to avoid unnecessary treatment. The neck may be successfully treated in approximately 60% of patients in whom clinically positive nodes appear and in whom the primary lesion remains controlled. However, even though the delayed neck treatment may be judged successful, these patients are at an increased risk of developing distant metastasis, because a positive lymph node that remains in the neck may act as a focus for dissemination to other lymph nodes or to distant sites. For patients presenting with a clinically negative neck, Jesse and coworkers (1970) reported an 11% incidence of distant metastasis in patients whose necks became positive compared with 3% for those whose necks remained controlled.

Strong (1979) reviewed patients with squamous cell carcinoma of the oral tongue managed by glossectomy and no elective neck treatment; 60% who developed neck disease died of uncontrolled cancer in the neck.

Harwood and coworkers (1983) reported that elective irradiation of the N0 neck for supraglottic larynx carcinomas decreased the incidence of neck failure from 29% to 4% and decreased tumor deaths from 35% to 5%.

Levendag and coworkers (1989) reported on 79 T1 N0 and T2 N0 squamous carcinomas of the supraglottic larynx. The death rate due to cancer was 0 (0%) of 56 patients whose necks remained controlled compared with 15 (65%) of 23 patients who relapsed in the neck.

In two separate multivariate analyses of patients with oral cavity cancer treated at the Royal Marsden Hospital or the Hopital Henri Mondor, it was found that the addition of elective neck treatment resulted in significantly improved survival rates compared with those of patients who had only follow-up of the neck and were treated upon relapse (Dearnaley et al. 1991; Piedbois et al. 1991).

Elective neck treatment is indicated, therefore, when the associated morbidity is low. It has the added advantage of giving complete treatment initially and simplifying the follow-up neck examinations because of its high success rate.

It can be easily demonstrated that elective neck treatment markedly reduces the subsequent appearance of neck disease. The effect on the overall survival rate is small, however, since approximately 60% of those who subsequently develop neck nodes are permanently salvaged. A randomized trial would require a large number of patients in order to detect a survival benefit. Although small randomized trials of elective neck treatment have been published (Fakih et al. 1989; Vandenbrouck et al. 1980), none to date have come close to including the numbers of patients needed to confirm or deny the survival advantage.

There is a large amount of data supporting the success of irradiation in eradicating subclinical disease in regional lymphatics. The control of subclinical disease increases with increasing dose; approximately 95% of subclinical lymph node metastases are controlled with 4500–5000 cGy over 5 weeks and 99% are controlled with 6000 cGy over 6 weeks. The common causes of failure of elective neck irradiation are geographic miss, low dose, and failure to detect an involved lymph node that is 1.5–2 cm or larger. Geographic miss or failure to adequately encompass all the lymph nodes at risk is the most common cause of failure and, at the University of Florida, occurred most often in oral tongue and floor of the mouth lesions when the primary portals were too small or when the low neck was not electively irradiated.

Low dose most often occurs when a lymph node is near the edge or corner of the portal (i.e., within 1–2 cm of the edge), and the dose may be 25% less than the dose in the central part of the treatment portal. The majority of so-called in-field failures result from the use of a portal that is slightly too small, which then creates a situation in which a lymph node near the margin receives less than the specified dose. Subclinical disease in a lymph node could range from a microscopic focus to a 1- to 1.5-cm node completely replaced by tumor, but clinically undetectable. The dose required to eliminate subclinical disease may be quite different at the extremes of tumor size. Fortunately, most positive lymph nodes occur in the first-echelon drainage area, which would receive 6000 cGy or more over 6 weeks as part of the treatment directed to the primary lesion.

If the primary lesion recurs, there is a renewed chance for lymphatic spread, and the neck is at considerable risk even if elective neck irradiation has been given.

Management of the Clinically Positive Neck

When the primary lesion is to be treated by radiation therapy only, irradiation alone is sufficient for patients with small N1 (1–2 cm) disease, but irradiation should sometimes be combined with a neck dissection for large N1 (3 cm) disease; neck dissection is almost always added following irradiation for N2a or N3a disease. For primary tumors of the nasopharynx, the neck nodes are more curable with irradiation alone.

The decision to add neck dissection for multiple ipsilateral nodes is individualized, based on the diameter of the largest node, the multiplicity of palpable nodes, and their distribution within the neck. For example, the neck may be staged N2b on the basis of a 2-cm subdigastric node and two 1-cm nodes in the upper neck; this neck might be treated with radiation therapy alone. Another patient with stage N2b might have small nodes located in the upper, mid, and lower neck and be better managed by adding neck dissection rather than administering a high dose to the entire neck. Yet another patient with N2b disease might have a 3- to 4-cm neck node and several other small nodes, and neck dissection should be considered.

Each side of the neck is considered separately when disease is bilateral; if possible, one side of the neck should be treated by irradiation alone. Bilateral neck dissections after radiation therapy may be staged or simultaneous. Most reports show a higher complication rate with simultaneous neck dissections, and the patient may require an elective tracheostomy, especially if the larynx has been irradiated. If enlarged nodes disappear completely and early during a course of radiation therapy, the likelihood of control by irradiation alone is improved and neck dissection may be withheld. However, if there is any question about complete regression, it is safer to add the neck dissection 4–8 weeks after radiation therapy, since the detection of neck node recurrence after high-dose radiation therapy is difficult and salvage attempts are generally morbid and unsuccessful. Mendenhall and coworkers (1986) reported only a 5% rate of successful salvage, and Bernier and Bataini (1986) reported a 1% success rate for the management of neck recurrence after irradiation alone for clinically positive neck nodes. Planned neck dissection 4–8 weeks after twice-daily radiotherapy (7400–8160 cGy) has been accomplished with acceptable morbidity and no operative mortality.

Radiotherapy alone for large-volume N2–N3 neck disease has several disadvantages:

1. The rate of disease control in the neck is poorer than when neck dissection is added.
2. Detection of recurrence is more difficult because of the fibrosis produced by both the high dose of radiotherapy and the fibrous reaction in and about the neck node.
3. Salvage surgery is infrequently successful after failure of radiotherapy alone and is accompanied by a relatively high incidence of wound complications (Mendenhall et al. 1984).
4. Paradoxically, the fibrosis produced in the soft tissues of the neck is actually greater in patients with large nodal masses who are cured by high-dose radiotherapy than in patients who receive similar doses of radiotherapy followed by radical neck dissection. In the former group, entrapment and paralysis of the 12th cranial nerve by dense fibrosis in the upper neck may occur, while it is rarely seen when a neck dissection is added. The explanation appears to be that the fibrous stroma of the lymph node itself contributes to overall fibrosis in the neck when it is not surgically removed.

When the primary lesion is to be treated by radiotherapy, our preference is that the neck dissection should follow radiotherapy. The advantages of this approach are several:

1. We have not considered it a good idea to perform neck dissection in the presence of an uncontrolled primary lesion, because surgical interruption of the lymphatics may lead to contralateral or bizarre patterns of lymph node metastasis due to collateral or aberrant flow (Fisch 1968).
2. For large lymph nodes, extranodal spread and fixation to the carotid sheath are rather common. After high-dose radiotherapy, the neck disease frequently becomes operable without carotid sacrifice.
3. If the neck dissection is performed before the radiotherapy, the radiotherapist then must "chase" surgical scars into areas that otherwise might not require treatment (e.g., into the submandibular region).

4. Performance of the neck dissection first leads to a delay in treating the primary site.
5. There is little published information to show the results of neck dissection when performed before radiation therapy of the primary site.
6. A scenario that sometimes occurs is that a patient with an unknown primary carcinoma is treated with a neck dissection before referral for irradiation. Under these circumstances, there is often postoperative edema of the ipsilateral hemilarynx, making the determination of the primary site difficult (e.g., pyriform sinus or supraglottic larynx).

Performance of radiotherapy first does have the disadvantage of potentially increasing the risk of severe surgical morbidity. A number of technical modifications, both radiotherapeutic and surgical, have been made through the years to minimize this problem. In our own series of patients, we believe that the risks of this treatment sequence are outweighed by the benefits. Large, fixed nodes (greater than 5–6 cm) may receive 6000–8000 cGy prior to neck dissection; one half of the specimens will show "no viable tumor," and quite a few patients will have the disease controlled in the neck.

Large lymph nodes may not show much regression during the course of the radiation treatments, but often show major change by the time the patient returns in 4–6 weeks for neck dissection. The node mass usually develops a thick capsule that facilitates dissection from the neurovascular bundle or other deep structures.

Management of the Neck After Excisional or Incisional Biopsy

Hayes Martin (Martin and Romieu 1952) and many who followed him taught that the injudicious biopsy of a cervical lymph node containing metastatic carcinoma for diagnosis before definitive therapy invariably lessened the chance for cure. In 1978, McGuirt and McCabe reviewed the University of Iowa experience for 64 patients who had a cervical node excised or incised before definitive treatment. Rates of neck recurrence, distant metastasis, and wound necrosis were significantly higher for the patients who had undergone neck biopsy compared with those who had no biopsy (605 patients) or had biopsy at the time of definitive therapy (46 patients). In their analysis, there were no data on the use of radiotherapy.

Parsons and colleagues (1985) reviewed the University of Florida experience for 80 patients who had an open biopsy of a cervical lymph node before definitive therapy and who were treated with radiation therapy as the initial treatment, followed in selected cases by neck dissection and in some cases by resection of the primary lesion. Regional control rates according to N-stage are shown in Table 1. The 5-year cause-specific survival rate for 17 evaluable patients with a single node excised and who were treated by radiation therapy was 88%. The 5-year cause-specific survival rates for those with gross residual neck disease were 32% for those treated by radiation

Table 1. Control of neck disease after neck node biopsy according to treatment technique with a minimum 2-year follow-up

N stage	Radiotherapy alone			Radiotherapy plus radical neck dissection		
	Treated (*n*)	Controlled		Treated (*n*)	Controlled	
		n	%		*n*	%
Nx	24	23	96	0	0	0
N1–N2	20[a]	13	65	7[b]	6	86
N3a	7	2	29	8	5	63

[a] Includes three N1, two N2a, and 15 N2b patients.
[b] Includes three N2a and four N2b patients.
(From Parsons et al. 1985)

therapy alone and 50% for those with a neck dissection added. These results were thought to be similar to those for stage III and IV patients without open biopsy, and it was concluded that radiation therapy should probably be the initial treatment after an open neck node biopsy; neck dissection and/or resection of the primary tumor should follow, depending on the clinical situation.

References

Bernier J, Bataini JP (1986) Regional outcome in oropharyngeal and pharyngolaryngeal cancer treated with high dose per fraction radiotherapy. Analysis of neck disease response in 1646 cases. Radiother Oncol 6:87–103

Dearnaley DP, Dardoufas C, A'Hearn RP, Henk JM (1991) Interstitial irradiation for carcinoma of the tongue and floor of mouth: royal Marsden Hospital experience 1970–1986. Radiother Oncol 21:183–192

Fakih AR, Rao RS, Borges AM, Patel AR (1989) Elective versus therapeutic neck dissection in early carcinoma of the oral tongue. Am J Surg 158:309–313

Fisch U (1968) Lymphography of the cervical lymphatic system. Saunders, Philadelphia

Harwood AR, Beale FA, Cummings BJ, Keane TJ, Payne DG, Rider WD, Rawlinson E, Elhakim T (1983) Supraglottic laryngeal carcinoma: an analysis of dose–time–volume factors in 410 patients. Int J Radiat Oncol Biol Phys 9:311–319

Jesse RH, Barkley HT Jr, Lindberg RD, Fletcher GH (1970) Cancer of the oral cavity: is elective neck dissection beneficial? Am J Surg 120:505–508

Levendag P, Sessions R, Vikram B, Strong EW, Shah JP, Spiro R, Gerold F (1989) The problem of neck relapse in early stage supraglottic larynx cancer. Cancer 63:345–348

Martin H, Romieu C (1952) The diagnostic significance of a "lump in the neck." Postgrad Med 11:491–500

McGuirt WF, McCabe BF (1978) Significance of node biopsy before definitive treatment of cervical metastatic carcinoma. Laryngoscope 88:594–597

Mendenhall WM, Million RR, Bova FJ (1984) Analysis of time–dose factors in clinically positive neck nodes treated with irradiation alone in squamous cell carcinoma of the head and neck. Int J Radiat Oncol Biol Phys 10:639–643

Mendenhall WM, Million RR, Cassisi NJ (1986) Squamous cell carcinoma of the head and neck treated with radiation therapy: the role of neck dissection for clinically positive neck nodes. Int J Radiat Oncol Biol Phys 12:733–740

Parsons JT, Million RR, Cassisi NJ (1985) The influence of excisional or incisional biopsy of metastatic neck nodes on the management of head and neck cancer. Int J Radiat Oncol Biol Phys 11:1447–1454

Piedbois P, Mazeron J-J, Haddad E, Coste A, Martin M, Levy C, Raynal M, Pavlovitch JM, Peynegre R, Pierquin B, Le Bourgeois JP (1991) Stage I–II squamous cell carcinoma of the oral cavity treated by iridium-192: is elective neck dissection indicated? Radiother Oncol 21:100–106

Strong EW (1979) Carcinoma of the tongue. Otolaryngol Clin North Am 12:107–114

Vandenbrouck C, Sancho-Garnier H, Chassagne D, Saravane P, Cachin Y, Micheau C (1980) Elective versus therapeutic radical neck dissection in epidermoid carcinoma of the oral cavity: results of a randomized clinical trial. Cancer 46:386–390

Radiotherapy with Different Fractionations and Simultaneous Cisplatin or Carboplatin in the Treatment of Advanced Head and Neck Carcinomas: Clinical Results and Radiobiological Investigations

T. Schnabel[1], N. Zamboglou[2], H. Bier[3], C.U. Fritzemeier[4], H. Bojar[5], E.T. Merholz[6], C. Kolotas[1], and G. Schmitt[1]

[1] Department of Radiation Oncology, Heinrich-Heine-University, Moorenstr. 5 40225 Düsseldorf, Germany
[2] Department of Radiation Oncology, Academic Hospital, Offenbach, Germany
[3] Department of ENT Surgery, Heinrich-Heine-University, Moorenstr. 5 40225 Düsseldorf, Germany
[4] Department of Maxillofacial Surgery, Heinrich-Heine-University Moorenstr. 5 40225 Düsseldorf, Germany
[5] Department of Chemical Oncology, Heinrich-Heine-University, Moorenstr. 5 40225 Düsseldorf, Germany
[6] Department of Maxillofacial Surgery, St. Lukas Clinic, Solingen, Germany

Introduction

Head and neck cancers can be treated with curative intent in the early stages by surgery or radiotherapy. Locally advanced carcinomas may not be controlled by single modality therapy, and local progression is the predominant cause of death. Radio-chemotherapy is gaining importance as primary treatment (Al-Sarraf 1988). Mitomycin-C, 5-fluorouracil (5-FU), bleomycin, methotrexate, and platinum derivatives have been used simultaneously with radiotherapy and have proven to be effective (Bachaud et al. 1991; Fu et al. 1987; Marcial et al. 1988; Sanchiz et al. 1990; Schnabel et al. 1991, 1992; Weissenberg et al. 1989; Wendt et al. 1988; Zamboglou et al. 1992). Unfortunately, some of these agents enhance mucosal reactions of concomitant radiotherapy (Fu et al. 1987; Wendt et al. 1988). In contrast, platinum derivatives do not enhance mucositis (Zambouglou et al. 1989, 1992). We report here on our experience using conventional and hyperfractionated, accelerated radiotherapy in combination with cisplatin and carboplatin in the management of advanced head and neck carcinomas as well as radiobiological investigations.

Cisplatin

From 1981 through 1987, advanced head and neck carcinomas were treated by a simple and well-tolerated regimen of radiotherapy and simultaneous cisplatin administration. A total of 111 patients with T2 N0–T4 N3 tumors of the oropharynx and oral cavity underwent this scheme. Of these, 53 had tumors of the oral cavity and 58 tumors of the oropharynx. All had biopsy-proven squamous cell carcinoma. The Tumor Node Metastasis (TNM) stage (UICC 1978) was T2 N1–3 in 11 patients, T3 N0–3 in 94, and T4 N0–3 in six patients. Radiotherapy was performed by means of a cobalt 60 unit or an 8 MeV linear accelerator up to a target absorbed dose of 40 Gy in a fractionation of 5 × 2 Gy/week. Cisplatin was given at a dose of 20 mg/m^2 during days 1–5 simultaneous to radiotherapy and hyperhydration. After a 2-week interval, tumor remission was evaluated. In case of a partial (PR) or complete remission (CR), radiotherapy was continued in a shrinking field technique up to a total dose of 70–74 Gy. A second course of cisplatin was given in week 7 over 5 days. Patients with tumors showing minor response after 40 Gy underwent interposed surgery and additional radiotherapy of 30 Gy and a second course of cisplatin. Forty-six patients had interposed surgery after 40 Gy.

Six weeks after the end of the whole treatment, 68 (67%) complete and 28 (27%) PR were achieved. The 5-year survival probability is 47% and is 6% higher in carcinomas of the oropharynx than in oral cavity cancers. In oropharyngeal cancer, survival curves of patients treated with radiotherapy alone or with interposed surgery did not show any difference. In contrast, radiotherapy alone achieved higher survival rates in oral cavity tumors than combined radiotherapy and interposed surgery. This may be ascribed to a negative selection of this group of patients.

Two patients developed esophageal variceal bleeding due to hyperhydration, and 95% had a temporary impairment of taste. Persistent taste impairment affected 21% of the patients who survived at least 1 year. Severe xerostomia occurred in 10% of all cases. Four percent developed osteoradionecrosis. Myelosuppression, transient renal toxicity, nausea, and vomiting were exceptional.

Carboplatin

Carboplatin is a second-generation platinum analog and has shown comparable antitumor activity to cisplatin in previous studies in patients with recurrent and metastatic head and neck tumors (Jacobs et al. 1989; Osoba et al. 1991; Schnabel et al. 1992; Zamboglou et al. 1989, 1992). The major difference between these compounds is their spectrum of side effects. The meta-analysis of three randomized trials comparing single-agent carboplatin and cisplatin in advanced ovarian cancer has shown that carboplatin induced significantly less nephrotoxicity, ototoxicity, neurotoxicity, and nausea/vomiting compared to cisplatin (Rozencweig et al. 1990). Carboplatin therapy does not require hyperhydration, but myelosuppression is more pronounced than with cisplatin. After having defined the maximum tolerable dose of carboplatin to be 70 mg/m^2 in a phase I study (Zamboglou et al. 1989), all patients with advanced head and neck cancers who embarked upon a phase II study (Zamboglou et al. 1992) were treated with two courses of carboplatin on days 1–5 and 29–33 and concomitant radiotherapy in a conventional fractionation of 5 × 2 Gy per week. The radiotherapy scheme was slightly modified compared to the cisplatin regimen insofar as a dose of 50 Gy was given before evaluating operability. This modification was made to overcome the tumor repopulation which is to be expected in the fourth week of radiotherapy (Withers 1985). From 1989 up to now, patients were treated with a dose of 60 mg/m^2, which resulted in a reduction of costs and myelotoxicity. This schedule can be performed on an outpatient basis.

Patients and Methods

From 1987 to 1991, 103 patients entered this protocol. A total of 100 patients have completed treatment so far and are eligible for tumor response and morbidity analysis. The median age was 57 years, ranging from 31 to 77 years. The median performance status World Health Organization (WHO) grade 2. Tumor stages and tumor sites are shown in Tables 1 and 2.

Carboplatin was given at a dose of 60 or 70 mg/m^2 i.v. over 30 min daily on days 1–5 and 29–33 before radiotherapy. A total of 56 patients received 70 mg/m^2 and 44 patients received 60 mg/m^2. After 50 Gy at 5 × 2 Gy/week and two courses of carboplatin, operability was evaluated with the help of the head and neck surgeons. Tumors showing a histopathologically complete remission after 50 Gy, two courses of carboplatin, and surgery did not receive an additional 20 Gy. Patients treated with radiotherapy alone received a total dose of 70–74 Gy.

Results

A total of 100 patients were evaluable. After 50 Gy and two cycles of carboplatin, only one patient showed a minor response. Thirty patients

Table 1. Tumor stage in carboplatin study (n = 100)

	T2	T3	T4
N0	2	5	4
N1	2	9	6
N2a	1	2	4
N2b	1	6	4
N2c	–	12	22
N3	–	5	15

Table 2. Tumor sites in carboplatin study ($n = 100$)

Tumor sites	No. of patients
Oral cavity	33
Oropharynx	8
Hypopharynx	7
Epipharynx	4
Larynx	3
Oral cavity/oropharynx	20
Oropharynx/hypopharynx	13
Hypopharynx/larynx	2
Epipharynx/oropharynx	3
Oropharynx/hypopharynx/larynx	1
Oropharynx/hypopharynx/epipharynx	1
Oral cavity/oropharynx/hypopharynx	3
Oropharynx/hypopharynx/Esophagus	1
Oropharynx/hypopharynx/larynx/Esophagus	1

underwent interposed surgery after 50 Gy, as directed by the surgeons. In eight of them, CR was confirmed by histopathological examination. The specimens of seven patients showed microscopic tumor residue, and in the others, macroscopic tumor residue was detected. The remaining 70 patients were treated with radiochemotherapy alone consisting of 70–74 Gy and two concomitant courses of carboplatin. In this group, tumor response was evaluated 6 weeks after the end of treatment. CR was achieved in 39 patients and PR in 30 patients. Only in one case was minor response seen. In summary, 69 patients were free of disease at the end of this combined treatment regimen.

The actuarial 1- and 2-year survival rates are 77% and 53%, respectively, for all patients. For patients with interposed surgery, the 1- and 2-year survival rates are 93% and 69%, and for the patients treated with radiotherapy alone, 71% and 47%, respectively. The differences between the curves are statistically significant, but one has to take into account that there was a positive selection of patients referred for interposed surgery. There was no significant difference between survival curves of patients with T3 and T4 tumors. However, the survival rate in patients with tumors involving only one compartment of the head and necks was significantly better than in patients having tumors involving two or more compartments (Fig. 1).

Toxicity

Leukopenia of WHO grades 3 and 4 occurred in nine and two out of 56 patients treated with 70 mg/m^2 carboplatin, respectively, and thrombocyto-

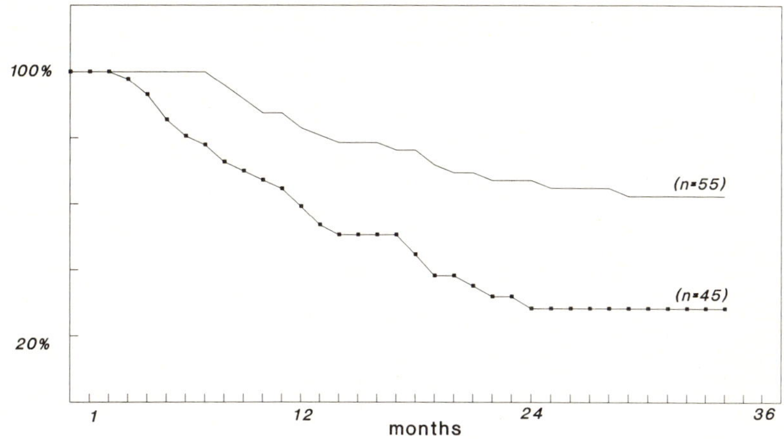

Fig. 1. Survival rates in patients with tumors involving one compartment (continous line) versus two or more compartments (boxed line) ($p < 0.05$)

penia of these degrees in four and three patients, respectively. A reduction to 60 mg/m^2 in the other 44 patients resulted in leukocytopenia grade 3 in one and grade 4 in another patient. Thrombocytopenia grade 3 was observed in three patients.

Radiobiological Investigations

Apart from clinical, prognostic factors, biological tests such as micronucleus formation, oncogenes, and DNA ploidy have been developed to individualize tumor treatment. DNA ploidy and micronucleus formation have been shown to give information on tumor biology, but are not yet integrated into clinical practice. We have analyzed 28 patients – 24 patients with T3 N2–3 carcinomas of the oral cavity and four patients with T3 N2 tumors of the oropharynx – using the following parameters: (a) fresh biopsies for flow cytometry, (b) paraffin-embedded specimens of the same patients for automated DNA-image cytometry. All patients received the same combined radiochemotherapy of 70–74 Gy in a conventional fractionation and two concomitant courses of cisplatin, as described above. Another group of 16 patients with T3 N3–T4 N2 tumors were irradiated with a hyperfractionated, accelerated split-course technique of twice-daily 1.6 Gy five times a week up to a target volume dose of 64–67.2 Gy (Karstens et al. 1989). Two courses of cisplatin were given simultaneously and the same biological tests were performed. After a minimum follow-up period of 2 years, 16 out of the 28 patients relapsed after conventional irradiation compared to seven of the group treated with hyperfractionated irradiation. Ploidy analysis showed a

5c ratio (i.e. ratio of cells with hyperpentaploidic DNA content) of the primary tumor in excess of 100/10 000 cells in 12 out of 16 patients. In contrast, only one out of 12 patients with a disease-free survival of more than 2 years had a 5c ratio exceeding 100/10 000 cells. The ploidy results of the group treated by accelerated hyperfractionation showed a 5c ratio exceeding 100/10 000 for 11 out of 16 patients, but only six of them developed recurrent tumor. This regimen seems to be more efficient than the classical form of radiotherapy in the treatment of head and neck carcinomas with a high proportion of hyperploid cells.

Hyperfractionated Accelerated Radiotherapy and Simultaneous Carboplatin Therapy

An optimal standard treatment regimen for advanced head and neck carcinomas has not yet been established. Simultaneous radiochemotherapy has achieved considerable local control rates in squamous carcinoma arising in the head and neck region (Glanzmann et al. 1990; Karstens et al. 1989; Sanchiz et al. 1990; Zamboglou et al. 1992). Apart from regimens using conventional fractionation radiotherapy, interest has focused on multiple daily fractionation to manage advanced disease (Wendt et al. 1988; Schnabel et al. 1992; Begg et al. 1992). A great variety of fraction numbers, doses per fraction, and overall treatment times have been reported (Barkley 1985; Cox et al. 1990; Glanzmann et al. 1990; Gray 1986; Karstens et al. 1989; Lamb et al. 1990; Marcial et al. 1988; Million et al. 1985; Osoba et al. 1991; Parsons et al. 1988; Sanchiz et al. 1990; Saunders et al. 1989; Schnabel et al. 1992; Volling et al. 1991; Wang et al. 1985, 1986; Wang 1989; Weissenberg et al. 1989; Wendt et al. 1988).

In order to evaluate the acute reactions and the therapeutic gain of hyperfractionated, accelerated radiotherapy and simultaneous carboplatin administration, a phase I feasibility study was initiated in 1990. Radiotherapy was performed according to a modified regimen reported by Wang et al. (1985) using a fractionation of 1.6 Gy twice a day up to a dose of 64–67.2 Gy, combined with two concomitant courses of Carboplatin.

Patients and Methods

Between 1990 and 1991, 15 patients with advanced head and neck carcinomas underwent hyperfractionated, accelerated radiotherapy and two courses of carboplatin. Eleven patients had T4 tumors and four had a T3 tumour. In six patients, lymph node involvement was staged as N3. Thirteen patients had two or more compartments of the head and neck involved.

All patients were irradiated with 1.6 Gy, two times a day, five times a week, with a minimum interval of 6 h between the fractions. Parallel opposed lateral fields were used up to a dose of 38.4 Gy. After a resting period of 8 days to allow acute radiation reaction to subside, fields were reduced to spare the spinal cord and the tumor dose was increased to 64 Gy using a shrinking field technique. In the case of macroscopic tumour residue, the total dose was raised to 67.2 Gy. With the exception of two patients (T3 N0, T3 N2b), all received 67.2 Gy. Carboplatin was administered at a dose of 60 mg/m^2 on days 1–5 and 29–33 of the treatment period.

Results

The median follow-up period is 10 months, with a range of 7–20 months. After the end of treatment, 12 patients had CR, and in the others PR was seen. All the PR patients died from tumor progression within 7 months, and one patient with CR succumbed 8 months after treatment. Eleven patients are still alive at 7–20 months (median: 10 months) with no evidence of disease. In two of these patients, salvage surgery was performed because of palpable residue, but CR was confirmed by histology. Ten patients developed a WHO grade 4 mucosal or dermal reaction at 28.8–38.4 Gy, which resolved after a rest period of 7–14 days. Five patients had a maximum grade 3 mucosal reaction. When treating the whole oral cavity, a rest period was often necessary at a dose of less than 38.4 Gy, as foreseen in the treatment schedule.

A leukopenia WHO grade 3 was seen in one patient, grade 2 in four, and grade 1 in one patient. In nine patients, leukocyte counts never dropped below 4000/μl during the treatment period. A thrombocytopenia WHO grade 1 was observed in two patients.

Discussion

Our results achieved with radiotherapy in combination with cisplatin are in good correlation with the results of other authors. Despite the fact that the schedule of cisplatin administration was different from that of the Radiation Therapy Oncology Group (RTOG)-81-17 protocol, the remission rate is comparable (Marcial et al. 1988). Mitomycin-C, 5-FU, methotrexate, and bleomycin have shown superior efficacy in the treatment of advanced head and neck carcinomas in combination with radiotherapy compared to radiotherapy alone (Fu et al. 1987; Sanchiz et al. 1990; Weissenberg et al. 1989). Cisplatin in combination with radiotherapy achieved better results even in a postoperative regimen of high-risk patients in a randomized study compared to irradiation alone (Bachaud et al. 1991). In order to develop a treatment of similar activity, but less toxicity, several phase I studies with carboplatin and simultaneous radiotherapy were carried out in patients with advanced head and neck carcinoma, achieving results comparable to those reported with cisplatin and cisplatin/5-FU regimens in combination with radiotherapy (Jacobs et al. 1989; Osoba et al. 1991). The CR rate of 69% induced by carboplatin plus radiotherapy is remarkable, considering that 45% of the tumors involved two or more regions of the head and neck and 55% were T4 tumors. Carboplatin with simultaneous radiotherapy in patients with inoperable head and neck carcinoma resulted in an antineoplastic activity comparable to cisplatin and cisplatin/5-FU-based regimens, but less non-hematologic toxicity. The results of calculating the biological efficacy of the two fractionation schemes used in our study are as follows: the biologically effective dose is 54.8 Gy for conventional and 54.0 Gy for hyperfractionated, accelerated irradiation, assuming that the cell doubling time is 5 days. In contrast, if the cell doubling time is thought to be 3 days, the biologically effective dose is 36 Gy for conventional and 47 Gy for hyperfractionated, accelerated irradiation. This might be an explanation for the increased efficacy of the hyperfractionation on hyperploid cells.

Multiple fractions per day are an essential feature of all recently designed, radiobiologically based, high-performance schedules, whether hyperfractionationed, accelerated, or both. Overall treatment time and dose per fraction operate differently on late- and early-reacting tissues, because cell proliferation in late-reacting tissues is slow or absent, but early-reacting tissues and tumors depend upon cells that proliferate rapidly. In late-reacting tissues, no compensatory proliferation occurs during a course of radiotherapy. The consequence is that overall time of radiotherapy can be doubled or halved with no change required in total dose and with no change in late complications if the total dose is not changed (Fowler 1989). On the other hand, prolonging overall treatment time means loss of tumor control. Both biological factors, overall treatment time, and dose per fraction seem to apply to the majority of tissues and tumors, so that new schedules can be planned that are effective in practice. The radiation schedule used by Parsons and coworkers (1988) consisted of two fractions of 1.2 Gy/day up to a total dose of 74.4–79.2 Gy. Local control of advanced tumours was improved by 10%–15% compared to another group previously treated with conventional fractionation in the same institution. A total of 20% of T4 lesions were controlled within a minimum follow-up period of 2 years. The authors defined mild complications as those which healed within 6 months of symptomatic treatment.

Other investigators used the European Organization for Research on Treatment of Cancer (EORTC)/RTOG or WHO staging system to assess side effects (Cox et al. 1990; Glanzmann et al. 1990; Sanchiz et al. 1990). In our study, side effects were obviously related to the treatment volume and were less severe and less frequent if the lips were not involved in the target volume. Wang et al. (1985, 1986; Wang 1989) reported improved local control rates of T3/T4 lesions of the oropharynx, larynx, and nasopharynx using a twice-daily fractionation consisting of 1.6 Gy/fraction up to a total dose of 64 Gy. Cox et al. (1990) used a fractionation of 1.2 Gy twice daily.

Patients were assigned to four groups receiving total doses between 67.2 and 76.8 Gy. There was a trend towards increased local control using doses in excess of 67.2 Gy, but no difference was observed in the survival rate.

Accelerated fractionation was used by Gray (1986) in a very heterogeneous group of advanced head and neck tumors. The overall local control rate was 52% in 48 patients treated with 1.8 Gy three times per day over 3 days a week. Acute reactions consisted of very brisk mucositis requiring skilled nursing care, but late tissue tolerance was entirely acceptable.

Karstens et al. (1989) achieved a complete tumor resolution in 12 out of 16 patients with stage III and IV head and neck carcinomas using our dose and fractionation regimen in combination with cisplatin. Unfortunately, the TNM staging and especially the lymph node involvement are not specified in this report. Because of the obligatory hyperhydration in cisplatinum regimens, patients with cardiac or renal disorders have to be excluded in favour of a carboplatin regimen.

Skov and Macphail (1991) have evaluated the interaction between radiation and carboplatin in vitro. The enhancement ratio of hypoxic cells was higher at low doses than at high doses. A longer incubation of tumor cells with carboplatin before irradiation markedly improved the interaction at low doses. This phenomenon might also influence the therapeutic efficacy of hyperfractionated radiotherapy with 1.6 Gy twice a day used in our study. In contrast to other studies (Cox et al. 1990; Glanzmann et al. 1990; Gray 1986; Million et al. 1985; Parsons et al. 1988), only one patient in our study had an AJCC (American Joint Commission on Cancer) stage III and fourteen patients had a stage IV disease. The initial complete remission rate of 80% for advanced tumors is unexpectedly high. Cox et al. (1990), Million et al. (1985), and Parsons et al. (1988) reported on lower local control rates in T4 lesions. The results of Karstens et al. (1989), Wendt et al. (1988), and Wang et al. (1985, 1986; Wang 1989) are in the same range. All patients with T4 tumors that entered our study had two or more compartments of the head and neck involved, which indicates a highly negative prognostic group. Twelve of the 15 patients also had an unfavorable involvement of the base of tongue. Because of the encouraging results achieved with hyperfractionated, accelerated radiotherapy, we initiated a multicenter, randomized study in November 1991. Patients with advanced head and neck carcinomas are either randomized for conventional radiotherapy with carboplatin or hyperfractionated, accelerated irradiation with carboplatin.

References

Al-Sarraf M (1988) Head and neck cancer: chemotherapy concepts. Semin Oncol: 70–85

Bachaud JM, David JM, Boussin G, Daly N (1991) Combined postoperative radiotherapy and weekly cisplatin infusion for locally advanced squamous cell carcinoma of the head and neck: preliminary report of a randomized trial. Int J Radiat Oncol Biol Phys 20:243–246

Barkley HT (1985) Accelerated treatment. Cancer 55:2112–2117

Begg AC, Hofland I, Van Glabekke M, Bartelink H, Horiot JC (1992) Predictive value of potential doubling time for radiotherapy of head and neck tumor patients: results from the EORTC cooperative trial 22851. Semin Radiat Oncol 2(1):22–25

Cox JD, Pajak TF, Marcial VA, Hanks GE, Mohiuddin M, Fu KK, Byhardt RW, Rubin P (1990) Dose-reponse for local control with hyperfractionated radiation therapy in advanced carcinomas of the upper aerodigestive tracts: preliminary report of radiation therapy oncology group protocol 83-13. Int J Radiat Oncol Biol Phys 18:515–521

Fowler JF (1989) The linear-quadratic formula and progress in fractionated radiotherapy. Br J Radiol 62:679–694

Fu KK, Philips TL, Silverberg IY (1987) Combined radiotherapy and chemotherapy with bleomycin and methotrexate for advanced inoperable head and neck cancer: update of a Northern California Oncology Group randomized trial. J Clin Oncol 5:1410–1418

Glanzmann C, Sartorelli B, Thum P, Lütolf UM (1990) Hyperfraktionierte Bestrahlung und simultane Chemotherapie mit Cisplatin bei Patienten mit fortgeschrittenen Karzinomen der Kopf-Hals-Region. Strahlenther Onkol 166:515–521

Gray AJ (1986) Treatment of advanced head and neck cancer with accelerated fractionation. Int J Radiat Oncol Biol Phys 12:9–12

Jacobs MC, Eisenberger M, Min Chuh Oh et al. (1989) Carboplatin and radiotherapy for stage IV carcinoma of the head and neck: a phase I–II study. Int J Radiat Oncol Biol Phys 17:361–369

Karstens JH, Hermes H, Schnarkowski P, Ammon J (1989) Accelerated fractionated irradiation with simultaneous cisplatin infusion in advanced head and neck cancer. Onkologie 12(4):187–189

Lamb DS, Spry NA, Gray AJ, Johnson AD, Alexander SR, Dally MJ (1990) Accelerated fractionation radiotherapy for advanced head and neck cancer. Radiother Oncol 18:107–116

Marcial V, Pajak TF, Kramer S et al. (1988) Radiation Therapy Oncology Group (RTOG) studies in head and neck cancer. Semin Oncol 15:39–60

Million RR, Parsons JT, Cassisi NJ (1985) Twice-a-day irradiation technique for squamous cell carcinomas of the head and neck. Cancer 55:2096–2099

Osoba D, Flores AD, Hay JH et al. (1991) Phase I study of concurrent carboplatin and radiotherapy in previously untreated patients with stage III and IV head and neck cancer. Head Neck 15:217–223

Parsons JT, Mendenhall WM, Cassisi NJ, Isaacs JH, Million RR (1988) Hyperfractionation for head and neck cancer. Int J Radiat Oncol Biol Phys 14:649–658

Rozencweig M, Martin A, Beitangandy M et al. (1990) Randomized trials of carboplatin versus cisplatin in advanced ovarian cancer. In: Bunn PA, Canetta R, Ozols RF et al. (eds) Carboplatin. Current perspectives and future directions. Saunders, Philadelphia, pp 175–186

Sanchiz F, Milla A, Torner J et al. (1990) Single fraction per day versus two fractions per day versus radio-chemotherapy in the treatment of head and neck cancer. Int J Radiat Biol Phys 19:1347–1350

Saunders MI, Dische S, Hong A et al. (1989) Continuous hyperfractionated accelerated radiotherapy in locally advanced carcinoma of the head and neck region. Int J Radiat Biol Phys 17:1287–1293
Schnabel TH, Zamboglou N, Daniel M, Schmitt G (1991) Treatment of advanced head and neck carcinomas in 101 patients with carboplatin and simultaneous irradiation. ECCO 6, Firenze, 27–31 Oct 1991
Schnabel TH, Zamboglou N, Kolotas C, Jimenez W, Strehl H, Schmitt G (1992) Phase I study of hyperfractionated accelerated radiation and simultaneous carboplatin therapy for advanced head and neck carcinomas. Strahlenther Onkol 168(6):318–321
Skov K, Macphail S (1991) Interaction of platinum drugs with clinically relevant X-ray doses in mammilian cells: a comparison of cisplatin, carboplatin, iproplatin, and tetraplatin. Int J Radiat Oncol Biol Phys 20:221–225
Volling P, Staar S, Achterrath W, Müller RP (1991) Carboplatin plus radiation therapy in head and neck cancer. Semin Oncol 18:17–22
Wang CC (1989) Accelerated hyperfractionation radiation therapy for carcinoma of the nasopharynx. Techniques and results. Canncer 63:2461–2467
Wang CC, Blitzer PH, Suit HD (1985) Twice-a-day radiation therapy for cancer of the head and neck. Cancer 55:2100–2104
Wang CC, Suit HD, Blitzer PH (1986) Twice-a-day radiation therapy for supraglottic carcinoma. Int J Radiat Biol Phys 12:3–7
Weissenberg JB, Son YH, Papac RJ, Sasaki C, Fischer D et al. (1989) Randomized clinical trial of mitomycin C as an adjunct to radiotherapy in head and neck cancer. Int J Radiat Oncol Biol Phys 17:3–9
Wendt TG, Wustrow TPU, Hartenstein RC, Trott KR (1988) Accelerated split-course radiotherapy and concomitant cisplatinum and 5-fluorouracil chemotherapy with folinic acid enhancement in unresectable head and neck cancer. Strahlenther Onkol 164:17–19
Withers HR (1985) Biologic basis for altered fractionation schemes. Cancer 55: 2086–2095
Zamboglou N, Pape H, Schnabel TH, Wurm R, Bannach B, Fürst G, Schmitt G (1989) Kombinierte Radiotherapie mit Cis- oder Carboplatin bei fortgeschrittenen Kopf-Hals-Tumoren. Strahlenther Onkol 165:647–651
Zamboglou N, Achterrath W, Schnabel TH, Lenaz L, Kolotas C, Schmitt G (1992) Simultaneous radiotherapy and chemotherapy with carboplatin in inoperable squamous cell carcinoma of the head and neck. A phase II study. Cancer Investigation 10(5):349–355

Curietherapy Versus External Irradiation Combined with Curietherapy in Stage II Squamous Cell Carcinomas of Mobile Tongue and Floor of Mouth

J.-J. Mazeron, L. Grimard, and V. Benk

Centre des Tumeurs, Hôpital La Salpêtrière, 47 Boulevard de l'Hôpital, 75013 Paris, France

Patients presenting with stage II squamous cell carcinomas (SCC) of mobile tongue and floor of mouth can be treated in many ways (Fletcher 1975; Pierquin et al. 1987). The management of these patients in France was routinely by interstitial irradiation to the primary area using iridium-192 and elective supraomohyoid neck dissection or close follow-up with delayed therapeutic neck dissection if required. The concept of elective irradiation of subclinical disease followed by an interstitial boost became very attractive in the mid-1970s and was used for tumors of the oral cavity (Fletcher 1972, 1975). This retrospective report describes our results with stage II SCC, comparing the two methods and paying special attention to local control.

Patients and Methods

From 1970 through 1986, 177 patients with stage II (UICC 1979) SCC of mobile tongue and floor of mouth were treated in the Department of Radiation Oncology at the Henri Mondor Hospital in Créteil, France. All patients were treated with curative intent. No patients were excluded from the analysis, irrespective of previous treatment, malignancy, or presence of synchronous primary, as the main objective of the review was to estimate local control by either approach. There were 157 males and 20 females. Their ages ranged from 31 to 84 years, with a mean of 58 years. The minimum follow-up was 3 years, and the maximum, 18 years. Patients were initially seen by a head and neck surgeon and a radiation oncologist. The clinical assessment included a full physical and ear, nose, and throat (ENT) examination with a direct laryngoscopy, an esophagoscopy, and a chest X-ray. All patients had a histologically proven SCC, and none had suspicious palpable nodes at presentation. The patients were staged retrospectively according to the Tumor Node Metastasis (TNM; UICC 1979) classification. The patients were further classified according to size of tumor: T2a if the

Table 1. Distribution of patients by treatment group

Tumor site	Group 1[a] (n = 132)	Group 2[b] (n = 45)
L	85	25
P	20	2
PL	19	13
PG	3	2
PLG	5	3
Tumor diameter		
T2a[c]	97	21
T2b[d]	35	24

L, lingual; P, pelvic; PL, pelvilingual; PG, pelvigingival; PLG, pelvilinguogingival. See text for details.
[a] Group 1, curietherapy alone.
[b] Group 2, external irradiation and interstitial boost.
[c] Less than or equal to 3 cm.
[d] Greater than 3 cm.

diameter was not more than 3 cm at any point or T2b if greater than 3 cm. The tumors were categorized according to their extension. Lesions involving the mobile tongue only were termed lingual (L); lesions involving the floor of mouth only were called pelvic (P); lesions arising from floor of mouth and involving the undersurface of the tongue were called pelvilingual (PL); lesions with extension from the floor of mouth to the gingiva were called pelvigingival (PG), and lesions with extension from the floor of mouth to the undersurface of the tongue and the gingiva were called pelvilinguogingival (PLG). The distribution of tumors by size and extension is shown in Table 1. The proportion of mobile tongue tumors was equivalent in group 1 (curietherapy alone) and group 2 (external irradiation and interstitial boost), being 64% (85 of 132) and 56% (25 of 47), respectively. By contrast, the proportion of T2a was greater in group 1 than in group 2, being 73% and 47%, respectively.

Treatment of the Primary

Most of the 132 patients included in group 1 were treated before 1975 or after 1980. The dose was prescribed, according to the Paris system, at the reference isodose corresponding to 85% of the basal dose rate (Dutreix et al. 1981; Pierquin et al. 1987). The basal dose rate is defined as the arithmetic mean of the minimum dose rates in the central transverse plane of the implant. The dose prescribed varied over the years in an attempt to improve the therapeutic ratio. It was 70 Gy from 1970 to 1975, was then reduced to 60 Gy, to be changed once more to 65 Gy in 1980. The reference dose rate (85% of the basal dose rate) varied from 0.3 Gy/h to 0.9 Gy/h. The techniques of interstitial therapy were the plastic tube or the guide gutter techniques previously described (Pierquin et al. 1987).

Patients included in group 2 were treated by a combination of external beam irradiation to the primary tumor and the regional lymphatics followed by an interstitial boost. Most of these patients were treated between 1975 and 1980 (Benk et al. 1990; Grimard et al. 1991). The patients were treated with cobalt 60 using two lateral portals covering the primary tumor and the neck. The fields extended from the base of skull superiorly to the hyoid bone inferiorly, and from the mandible symphysis anteriorly to the tip of the spinal processes posteriorly. Those portals were matched with an anterior field to treat the lower neck and the supraclavicular nodes with midline shielding of the larynx and spinal cord plus shielding of the pulmonary apices. The usual dose was 45 Gy, given in fractions of 1.8 Gy five times per week. External beam irradiation was followed by implantation of the primary to deliver an additional 30 Gy to the initial tumor volume plus safety margin as with brachytherapy alone.

The interstitial dose was calculated using the "escargot curve" from orthogonal films and a tomographic view in the transverse plane of the implant from 1970 to 1976. The "escargot" is a graphic template to estimate dose rates directly on a diagrammatic reconstruction of the source pattern (Dutreix et al. 1981). Computerized dosimetry was introduced in 1976 and used routinely thereafter.

Neck Management

For patients in group 1, the neck was managed by an elective neck dissection, consisting of bilateral supraomohyoid dissection that was extended when metastasic nodes were found and followed by postoperative irradiation of up to 55 Gy with shielding of the volume previously implanted (Piedbois et al. 1991). The spinal cord dose was limited to 45 Gy by using electrons. In the late 1970s, the patients were either followed closely or had an elective neck dissection, based on the results from a randomized study showing no difference in survival (Vandenbrouck et al. 1980). Patients who suffered neck relapses underwent, when feasible, a functional or a radical neck dissection, followed by postoperative irradiation of up to 55 Gy. The previously implanted volume was shielded such that the rami and the lower half of the body of the mandible were in the external beam and the alveolar process of the mandible was shielded. Seventy-eight patients had an elective neck dissection and 54 patients were closely followed. For patients in group 2, the neck was managed by elective irradiation of up to 45 Gy.

Results

Floor of Mouth

The 5-year survival rate was 35% for the entire population, and there was no difference between the two treatment groups. The proportion of deaths from disease and treatment was the same in both groups, being 32% and 30%, respectively (Grimard et al. 1991).

The primary local control was 73%, and salvage surgery was successful in three patients for an ultimate local control of 78%. There was no difference between both groups, as shown in Table 2. The poor local control of patients with gingival extension is summarized in Table 3. There were local failures in seven out of 13 patients (53%) in the group with gingival extension, and in 11 out of 54 (20%) in the group without gingival extension ($p < 0.04$).

Fourteen patients developed a neck recurrence. It was associated with primary tumor failure in nine patients: six in group 1 and three in group 2. None of these nine locoregional failures were salvaged. There was no isolated neck recurrence in group 2 and five in group 1: two among the 23 patients with negative neck dissection (both necks were salvaged) and three among the 14 patients with close follow-up (one was salvaged and two died

Table 2. Floor of mouth cancers: local control according to treatment policy

	Group 1[a] (n = 47)	Group 2[b] (n = 20)
Before salvage	35 (74%)	14 (70%)
After salvage	37 (79%)	15 (75%)

[a] Group 1, curietherapy alone.
[b] Group 2, external irradiation and interstitial boost.

Table 3. Floor of mouth cancers: local control according to gingival extension

	Group 1[a] (n = 47)	Group 2[b] (n = 32)
P + PL	32/39 (82%)	11/15 (73%)
PG + PLG	3/8	3/5

P, pelvic; PL, pelvilingual; PG, pelvigingival; PLG, pelvilinguogingival.
[a] Group 1, curietherapy alone.
[b] Group 2, external irradiation and interstitial boost.

of neck failures). One patient died following an elective neck dissection. Three patients died of neck disease and/or treatment in group 1.

There were two deaths attributed to treatment; one from an elective neck dissection (already mentioned) and one postoperative death following a partial mandibulectomy and reconstruction for a radiation-induced osteoradionecrosis. Both deaths occurred in group 1 patients.

Radionecrosis was grade I when patients did not require more than ambulatory conservative treatment and the necrosis healed within 6 months, grade II when necrosis required a hospital admission for intensive treatment, usually consisting of antibiotics and steroids, and grade III when the radiation-induced complications required surgical intervention, minor or major, or when debilitating, persistent sequelae or death occurred. There were 16 soft tissue sequelae and ten bone complications. There were 11 grade I (ten patients), six grade II (five patients), and nine grade III (five patients, including one death) complications.

Mobile Tongue

The 5-year survival rate was 38% for the entire group. It was 49% for the T2a patients and 20% for the T2b patients. Sixteen percent of patients with T2a tumors died of disease, compared with 46% of patients with T2b tumors ($p < 0.01$; Benk et al. 1990). The 5-year survival rate was 42% in group 1 (curietherapy alone) versus 24% in group 2 (external irradiation and interstitial boost). Twenty percent of patients died of disease in group 1 versus 52% in group 2 ($p < 0.01$). A comparison of survival rates between the two groups is of limited use because of the unequal distribution by size, as shown in Table 1. Causes of death and survival are displayed by tumor size and treatment policy in Table 4.

Table 4. Mobile tongue cancers: 5-year survival and causes of death

	Group 1[a]		Group 2[b]	
	T2a (n = 51)	T2b (n = 20)	T2a (n = 6)	T2b (n = 15)
Survival	26 (51%)	4 (20%)	2 (33.3%)	3 (20%)
Causes of death				
T ± N ± M	2	4	2	8
N ± M	4	3		
M	1			1
Intercurrent	10	6		3
Unknown	6	2	2	
Lost of follow-up	2	1		

T, tumor; N, node; M, metastasis.
[a] Group 1, curietherapy alone.
[b] Group 2, external irradiation and interstitial boost.

Table 5. Mobile tongue cancers: local control

	Group 1[a] T2a (n = 63)	T2b (n = 22)	Group 2[b] T2a (n = 8)	T2b (n = 25)
Primary control	90%	82%	47.5%	35%
After salvage	95%	82%	50%	44%

[a] Group 1, curietherapy alone.
[b] Group 2, external irradiation and interstitial boost.

Table 6. Mobile tongue cancers: neck control

	Group 1[a] T2a (n = 59)	T2b (n = 21)	Group 2[b] T2a (n = 6)	T2b (n = 15)
Before salvage				
Primary controlled	47/53	10/17	2/2	3/4
Primary not controlled	5/6	4/4	2/4	8/11
After salvage				
Primary controlled	52/53	12/17	2/2	3/4
Primary not controlled	5/6	4/4	2/4	8/11

[a] Group 1, curietherapy alone.
[b] Group 2, external irradiation and interstitial boost.

The primary control was significantly better in patients treated exclusively by interstitial therapy: 88% in group 1 compared to 46% in group 2 ($p < 0.01$). The difference in local control was still present after correction for tumor size. Salvage surgery, attempted in five patients, was successful in three of the 26 local recurrences. Local control by tumor size and treatment group is shown in Table 5. Local control in group 1 patients, excluding two patients treated by more than one implant, was obviously dose dependent, being 80% for doses less than 63 Gy compared to 92% for 63 Gy or more ($p = 0.11$; Benk et al. 1990; Mazeron et al. 1990b; Mendenhall et al. 1989).

Patients who died of intercurrent disease or unknown cause within 2 years of treatment and those lost to follow-up were excluded from the regional control analysis, leaving 101 of the 110 patients. Neck control was 94% for T2a patients and 75% for T2b patients after salvage ($p < 0.01$). Nodal failures were more common when the primary tumor was not controlled. There were, after salvage, seven isolated neck failures among the 76 patients with the primary controlled (9%), compared to six among the 25 patients with uncontrolled tumor (24%). Definitive regional control was 91% in group 1 versus five out of six in group 2 when the primary site was controlled. No significant difference was seen in group 1 patients according to neck management. Definitive regional control was 89% in patients having an

Table 7. Mobile tongue cancers; necroses (84 patients at risk)

Grade[a]	Grade 1	Grade 2	Grade 3
Soft tissue	11	2	1
Bone	12	1	3

[a] See text for details.

elective neck dissection and 77% in patients having surveillance with therapeutic neck dissection and irradiation for relapse. Regional control by tumor size and treatment group is summarized in Table 6.

The rate of necrosis after excluding patients with local recurrence is given in Table 7. No significant difference was seen for soft tissue or bone necrosis by treatment category, being one and two out of nine patients in group 2 compared to 13 and 14 out of 75 patients in group 1, respectively. Four patients required corrective surgery for radionecrosis; three of these were from group 2.

Discussion

The concept of eradicating subclinical disease (disease present, but not clinically detectable) with a 90% probability following 45–50 Gy over 5 weeks was attractive in the management of stage II tumors of the oral cavity. Following the publication of encouraging results by Fletcher (1972, 1975), the policy of external beam irradiation followed by an interstitial boost was attempted in many French centers. A common result was a dramatic reduction in primary control, such that this approach was discontinued in most centers in the early 1980s.

Among 147 T2 N0 patients with SCC of the mobile tongue, Pernot et al. (1992) observed, a 5-year local control of 89.8% (70 patients) when treated by curietherapy alone versus 50.6% (77 patients) when external beam irradiation was combined with an interstitial boost, with a difference in cause-specific survival of 62.2% versus 34.7% at 5 years. Our team had the same experience in the present series, with a primary control of 88% versus 36% with these treatments. These results were very similar for different European Groups (Haie et al. 1983), as expressed at the meeting of the Groupe Européen de Curiethérapie in Sitges, Spain, in 1988. A recent review from the M.D. Anderson Hospital on 85 stage II oral tongue cancers treated from 1963 to 1979 showed a better local control rate when the dose delivered by brachytherapy using radium needles was moderately high and the external beam component was less than 40 Gy: 92% versus 64% (Wendt et al. 1990). The same phenomenon was observed at the University of Florida (Mendenhall et al. 1989).

Another purpose of the present review was to see if local control would also be different according to treatment policy in stage II SCC of the floor of mouth. There are few data on the subject and none on patients treated during the same period by the same physicians as in our series. The small number of patients in group 2 (20 patients) would allow only major differences to be detected; none were seen. Does one treatment policy offer a better chance of cure over the other? This question could be answered through a prospective randomized trial comparing both approaches in the management of stage II SCC of the floor of mouth.

The use of combined external irradiation and interstitial boost for stage II SCC of mobile tongue and floor of mouth was discontinued in 1979 in our center (Benk et al. 1990; Mazeron et al. 1990). Currently, patients with T2 N0 SCC are managed by curietherapy alone at a dose of up to 65–70 Gy, using the Paris system. Management of the neck remains an unresolved problem. Patients are either observed or undergo an elective supraomohyoid neck dissection, according to individual physician's preferences, previous neck treatment, and whether close follow-up is realistic in individals whose life-style is frequently anything but health conscious. Patients with lesions extending to the gingiva (PG and PLG) are managed by surgery in the majority of cases (Mazeron et al. 1990; Grimard et al. 1991).

The high complication rate from interstitial irradiation previously found is no longer a problem when modern techniques of brachytherapy are used and patients are properly selected. Ideally, the latter condition is optimized in a multidisciplinary clinic where surgeon and radiation oncologist jointly assess each new patient. The risk of clinically significant complications from curietherapy under these conditions is small and quite acceptable. The introduction of individualized intraoral mandibular shields, not used in this series, has reduced even further the risk of osteoradionecrosis. Cosmetic and functional results (particularly concerning speech) are optimal, and xerostomia is avoided.

Conclusion

For patients with a mobile tongue stage II SCC, this retrospective analysis shows better results in patients whose primary was treated by interstitial irradiation alone. Accelerated repopulation of clonogenic malignant cells may represent the main reason why a protracted course of external beam irradiation followed by an interstitial boost gave poor results. For patients with a floor of mouth stage II SCC, no major difference was seen between those whose primary tumor was treated with interstitial curietherapy alone and those treated with a combination of external beam irradiation and curietherapy. Curietherapy alone is preferred as it preserves salivary function and is recommended for lesions without gingival extension. The problem of subclinical regional disease remains unresolved. The neck could be managed either by an elective bilateral supraomohyoid dissection, extended when metastatic nodes are found, plus a postoperative irradiation to a dose of 55 Gy with shielding of the previously implanted volume, or by a policy of close surveillance with delayed therapeutic dissection and radiotherapy.

References

Benk V, Mazeron JJ, Grimard L, Crook J, Haddad E, Piedbois P, Raynal M, Martin M, Le Bourgeois JP, Pierquin B (1990) Comparison of curietherapy versus external irradiation combined with curietherapy in stage II squamous cell carcinomas of the mobile tongue. Radiother Oncol 18:339–347

Dutreix A, Marinello G, Wambersie A (1981) Dosimétrie en curiethérapie. Masson, Paris

Fletcher GH (1972) Elective irradiation of subclinical disease in cancers of the head and neck. Cancer 19:1450–1454

Fletcher GH (1975) Textbook of radiotherapy, 2nd edn. Lea and Febiger, Philadelphia

Grimard L, Mazeron JJ, Pierquin B (1991) Comparison of curietherapy versus external irradiation combined with curietherapy in stage II squamous cell carcinomas of the floor of mouth. Endocur Hypertherm Oncol 7:97–103

Haie C, Gerbaulet A, Wibault P, Chassagne D, Marandas P (1983) Résultats de la curiethérapie et de l'association radiothérapie transcutanée-curiethérapie dans 155 cancers de la langue mobile. Expérience de l'Institut Gustave Roussy. Actual Carcinol Cervico Faciale 9:53–57

Mazeron JJ, Crook J, Benk V, Marinello G, Martin M, Raynal M, Haddad E, Peynegre R, Le Bourgeois JP, Walop W, Pierquin B (1990a) Iridium implantation for T1 and T2 epidermoid carcinoma of the mobile tongue: the Créteil experience. Int J Radiat Oncol Biol Phys 19:1369–1376

Mazeron JJ, Crook JM, Marinello G, Wallop W, Pierquin B (1990b) Prognostic factors of local outcome for T1, T2 carcinomas of oral tongue treated by iridium 192 implantation. Int J Radiat Oncol Biol Phys 19:281–285

Mazeron JJ, Grimard L, Raynal M, Haddad E, Piedbois P, Martin M, Marinello G, Nair RC, Le Bourgeois JP, Pierquin B (1990c) Iridium 192 curietherapy for T1 and T2 epidermoid carcinomas of the floor of mouth. Int J Radiat Oncol Biol Phys 18:1299–1306

Mazeron JJ, Simon JM, Le Péchoux C, Crook JM, Grimard L, Piedbois P, Le Bourgeois JP, Pierquin B (1991) Effect of dose rate on local control and complications in definitive irradiation of T_{1-2} squamous cell carcinomas of mobile tongue and floor of mouth with interstitial iridium 192. Radiother Oncol 21:39–47

Mendenhall WM, Parsons JT, Stringer SP, Cassisi NJ, Million RR (1989) T2 oral tongue carcinoma treated with radiotherapy: analysis of local control and complications. Radiother Oncol 16:275–281

Pernot M, Malissard L, Aletti P, Hoffstetter S, Forçard JJ, Bey P (1992) Iridium-192 brachytherapy in the management of 147 T2N0 oral tongue carcinomas treated with irradaiation alone: comparison of two treatment techniques. Radiother Oncol 23:223–228

Piedbois P, Mazeron JJ, Haddad E, Coste A, Levy C, Raynal M, Pavlovitch JM, Peynegre R, Pierquin B Le Bourgeois JP (1991) Stage I–II squamous cell carcinoma of the oral cavity treated by iridium 192: is elective neck dissection indicated? Radiother Oncol 21:100–107

Pierquin B, Wilson F, Chassagne D (1987) Modern Brachytherapy. Masson, New York

UICC: Union Internationale Contre le Cancer (1979) Tumor Node Metastasis (TNM) classification of tumors, 3rd edn. UICC, Geneva

Vandenbrouck C, Sancho-Garnier H, Chassagne D, Saravane D, Cachin Y, Micheau C (1980) Elective versus therapeutic radical neck dissection in epidermic carcinoma of the oral cavity: results of a randomized clinical trial. Cancer 46:386–390

Wendt CD, Peters LJ, Delclos L, Ang KK, Morrison WH, Maor MH, Robbins KT, Byers RM, Carlson LS, Oswald MJ (1990) Primary radiotherapy in the treatment of stage I and II oral tongue cancers: importance of the proportion of therapy delivered with interstitial therapy. Int J Radiat Oncol Biol Phys 18:1287–1292

Present Status of EORTC Trials of Hyperfractionated and Accelerated Radiotherapy on Head and Neck Carcinoma

J.C. Horiot[1], A.C. Begg[2], R. Le Fur[3], S. Schraub[4], W. van den Bogaert[5], M. van Glabbeke[6], and M. Pierart[6]

[1] Tumor Institute Centre G.F. Leclerc, 1 rue du Professeur Marion, 21034 Dijon, France
[2] Tumor Institute A. van Leeuwenhoekhuis, Plesmanlaan 121, 1066 CX Amsterdam, The Netherlands
[3] Tumor Institute Centre H. Becquerel, rue d'Amiens, 76038 Rouen, France
[4] University Hospital Jean Minjoz, Boulevard Fleming, 28000 Besançon, France
[5] University Hospital Sint Rafael, Capucijnenvoer 33, 3000 Leuven, Belgium
[6] European Organization for Research on Treatment of Cancer Data Centre, 83 avenue E. Mounier, 1260 Brussels, Belgium

Introduction

The European Organization for Research on Treatment of Cancer (EORTC) Cooperative Group of Radiotherapy started phase II and III trials on modified fractionation schemes in 1980. As of June 1, 1992, 2006 patients have entered eight trials. This short overview will only concentrate on two phase III trials of hyperfractionation (EORTC trial 22791) and accelerated fractionation (trial 22851).

Pure hyperfractionation (HF) is defined as an increased number of fractions, using a smaller dose per fraction, delivered over the same overall treatment time as in conventional fractionation (CF). Withers and Horiot 1987). The objective of our investigation was to evaluate the normal tissue tolerance and results in using two fractions versus one fraction per day. The fraction size investigated was 1.15 Gy. The minimum interval between two daily fractions was 4 h at the beginning of the study and was extended to about 8 h in 1985.

In accelerated fractionation (AF), the overall treatment time is shorter than in CF. This was achieved by using three fractions per day with 4 h between the daily fractions, aiming at the same total dose as in CF and shortening the overall treatment time by at least 2 weeks.

Hyperfractionation

The EORTC trial 22791 consisted in a phase III study of two fractions of 1.15 Gy per day (total dose 80.5 Gy in 70 fractions over 7 weeks) versus a single daily fraction of 2 Gy (total dose 70 Gy in 35 fractions over 7 weeks).

Patients with oropharyngeal carcinoma staged T2 or T3, N0 or N1 <3 cm, and M0 were randomized to one of these two arms. The use of two fractions per day offers the best interval between fractions (about 8 h) during an 8-h working day, thus allowing normal tissue to repair most of the sublethal damage between fractions. A pilot study of 103 patients (Horiot et al. 1982) established that a 15% higher dose per day could be delivered to the target volume. The question addressed by the present trial was whether the same increase in total dose would be sufficient to improve locoregional control (LRC) without increasing late morbidity.

Patients and Methods

The selection of patients included T2 and T3 N0 or N1 of less than 3 cm oropharyngeal squamous cell carcinoma (except for primaries arising from the base of the tongue). Patients were randomized either to the CF (70 Gy in 35 fractions over 7 weeks) or the HF arm (80.5 Gy in 70 fractions over 7 weeks). The dose to the spinal cord was to be kept below 50 Gy in the two arms. From 1980 to 1987, 356 patients entered the trial at 28 institutions from seven European countries. Ninety percent of the patients are fully evaluable for the final analysis.

Acute and Late Tolerance

Objective acute tolerance based upon the scoring of acute mucosal reactions was decreased in the HF arm ($p = 0.01$), resulting in a prolongation of the overall treatment time in 13% of the patients and precluding that the prescribed dose be reached in only 6%. Late damage to normal tissue was evaluated with an actuarial estimate of the absence of grade 2 and 3 late tissue damage (Fig. 1). No difference is observed between the two treatment arms, thus confirming the accuracy of the radiobiological prediction for normal tissue tolerance in the head and neck area. These results are of particular interest for more slowly proliferating normal tissue such as bone and connective tissues.

Locoregional Control

The 5-year LRC is significantly higher ($p = 0.01$) in the HF arm than in the CF arm (56% versus 38%) (Fig. 2). This advantage was only observed in the 217 patients with a good initial performance status (Karnovsky index of 90–100). The superiority of the HF regime was also demonstrated in patients staged T3 N0 or T3 N1, but not T2. The Cox model confirmed that the treatment regime was an independently significant prognostic factor for LRC ($p = 0.007$).

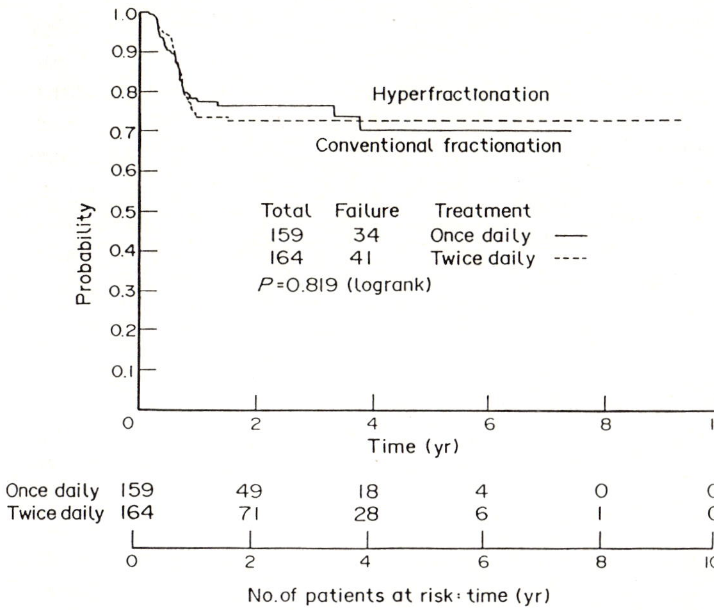

Fig. 1. Probability of avoiding late side effects of grade 2 or 3 (EORTC trial 22791)

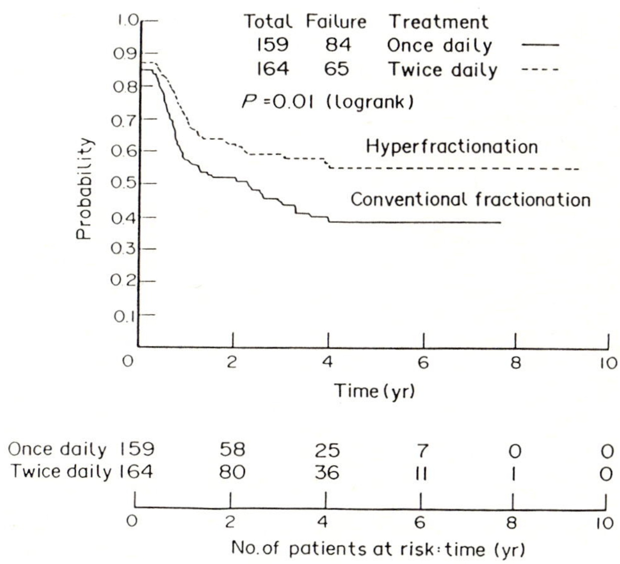

Fig. 2. Probability of remaining free of locoregional disease (EORTC trial 22791)

Survival

Survival was not an end point in this study, due to the significant risk of death from other cancers and from intercurrent disease in this population of patients. However, the improvement of LRC was responsible for a trend towards an improved 5-year survival rate ($p = 0.07$).

Comments

This is the first controlled clinical trial to provide evidence of the benefit of delivering two fractions per day instead of one. The trial also stresses the importance of selecting patients in good general condition and with moderately advanced tumors to assess the potential improvements of new radiotherapy regimes in head and neck carcinoma.

Accelerated Fractionation

The EORTC trial 22851 consisted in a phase III study of AF in the radiotherapy of advanced head and neck carcinoma. After stratification, patients were randomized either to the conventional regime (single fraction per day of 1.8–2 Gy for 7–8 weeks; total dose 70 FGy in 35 fractions over 7 weeks to 72 Gy in 40 fractions over 8 weeks) or to the AF regime of three fractions of 1.6 Gy per day described below. The rationale underlying the protocol is based upon the following objectives: (a) to reduce the overall treatment time by 2 weeks (e.g., from 7 to 5 weeks), (b) to maintain a total dose equal to the total dose planned in CF, and (c) to ensure an acceptable mucosal tolerance during the treatment in order to complete it prior to the peak of acute mucosal reactions. Previous pilot studies from Dijon and Leuven using multiple fractions per day (three fractions of 1.6 Gy with 4 h between the fractions) with increasing doses delivered in the first course of treatment demonstrated a steep dose response – in terms of acute mucosal reactions – between 24 Gy over 5 days in 15 fractions and 33.6 Gy over 8 days in 21 fractions. The lower dose was consistent with a moderate mucositis and a rapid recovery, while the higher dose was almost always associated with grade 3 mucositis and a longer recovery time. It soon appeared that it was essential not to interfere with normal tissue repopulation during the second week after the start of treatment. Hence, the first sequence of the AF regime in the trial consisted of 28.8 Gy over 7 days in 18 fractions. The second course started on day 21 using the same fractionation schedule. It delivered 43.2 Gy in 27 fractions over 11 days to a cumulative dose of 72 Gy in 45 fractions over 4.5–5 weeks for the two treatment courses. The dose to the spinal cord was kept below 36 Gy in 5 weeks in the AF arm and below 50 Gy in 7 weeks in the CF arm.

Status of the Trial

From 1985 to June, 1, 1992, 410 patients entered the trial in 22 institutions. The trial is still going on (aiming at a total accrual of 500 patients). Hence, it is not yet possible to disclose the interim analysis per treatment arm, and we shall review only the observed acute and late toxicities.

Acute Toxicity (Table 1)

A total of 257 patients are fully evaluable (122 in the CF arm and 135 in the AF arm) for functional and objective mucosal reactions up to 6 weeks after the end of radiotherapy. There is a highly significant increase in the acute toxicity in the AF arm, although this did not interfere with the completion of the prescribed treatment, since the worst reactions always occur within a few days of treatment completion.

Severe Late Toxicity

Ten patients (2.4%) died from a treatment-induced complication; eight out of ten were treated in the AF arm. Deterioration of general condition during treatment and denutrition without recovery were observed in five cases (four in the AF arm) and were the main reasons for death from complications in the first 8 months (other reasons included mucosal ulcers

Table 1. European Organization for Research on Treatment of Cancer (EORTC) trial 22851: maximum score of acute mucositis up to 6 weeks after the end of radiotherapy

	Grade		CF arm	AF arm	Total
Functional mucosal reaction	0	No complaints	19 (15.6%)	5 (3.7%)	24 (9.3%)
	1	Mild irritation	17 (13.9%)	9 (6.7%)	26 (10.1%)
	2	Moderate, irritation	37 (30.3%)	28 (20.7%)	65 (25.3%)
	3	Liquid diet only	37 (30.3%)	52 (38.5%)	89 (34.6%)
	4	Alimentation impossible	5 (4.1%)	38 (28.1%)	43 (16.7%)
	9	Unevaluable	7	3	10
		Total	122 (100%)	135 (100%)	257 (100%)
Objective mucosal reaction	0	No mucosal reaction	18 (14.8%)	6 (4.4%)	24 (9.3%)
	1	Mild mucositis	24 (19.7%)	6 (4.4%)	30 (11.7%)
	2	Patchy mucositis	30 (24.6%)	22 (16.3%)	52 (20.2%)
	3	Diffuse mucositis	43 (35.2%)	97 (71.9%)	140 (54.5%)
	9	Unevaluable	7	4	11
		Total	122 (100%)	135 (100%)	257 (100%)

AF, accelerated fractionation; CF, conventional fractionation.

Table 2. European Organization for Research on Treatment of Cancer (EORTC) trial 22851: causes of death (interim analysis March 1992)

Cause of death	No. of patients
Malignant disease	102
Complication of treatment	10
Cardiovascular disease	8
Associated chronic disease[a]	4
Second primary tumor	7
Other[b]	8
Unknown	8
Infection	4
Total	151

[a] One severe chronic bronchitis, one gastroduodinal ulcer (postoperative death), one alcoholic cirrhosis, and one liver decompensation.
[b] One intercurrent cardiorespiratory accident, two intercurrent deaths (drowning and car accident), one murder, one acute pancreatitis, one hemorrhage, one epilepsy, and one diffuse cerebral anoxia.

and hemorrhages). Death from complications after 1 year consisted of another mucosal necrosis at 14 months and a brain necrosis at 27 months in a patient treated for a nasopharyngeal carcinoma. A single case of transverse myelitis was observed in the AF arm with a spinal cord dose of 36 Gy over 5 weeks.

Status of Patients

A total of 151 patients (37%) have already died; causes of death are listed in Table 2. Unfortunately, the cell kinetics parameters were only obtained 1 year after the start of trial and were not mandatory. As from April 1991, it was decided to record this information in all patients.

Results

Cell kinetics parameters were obtained from biopsies performed about 6 h after an i.v. injection of 100 mg/m^2 iodo-deoxyuridine (IUdR) and analyzed with flow cytometry by Begg et al. (1985, 1990). The IUdR was obtained from the National Cancer Institute in Bethesda, USA, as a freeze-dried powder and dissolved with sterile water. Due to the time required to obtain approval for use of IUdR in this trial, no patients were labeled in the first

Table 3. Mean and variation of cell kinetic parameters in head and neck tumors measured by iodo-deoxyuridine and flow cytometry

	Mean	SD	CV (%)	Minimum	Maximum
T_s	11.2	4.4	39	4.8	33.2
LI	12.7	6.0	47	2.4	30.5
T_{pot}	4.7	3.2	68.5	1.4	16.9

SD, standard deviation (n = 68); CV, coefficient of variation; T_s, DNA synthesis time; LI, labeling index; T_{pot}, cell cycle time divided by the proportion of cells in cycle.

year of the trial. The success rate for obtaining analyzable cell kinetic data from the biopsy material was 85%. A summary of values for the pretreatment cell kinetic parameters DNA synthesis time (T_s), labeling index (LI), and cell cycle time divided by the proportion of cells in cycle (T_{pot}) is given in Table 3. For each parameter, there was a wide range of values, being greatest for T_{pot} (coefficient of variation, 69%) with mean and median values of 4.7 and 3.8 days, respectively. T_s was not significantly correlated with LI. The influence of T_{pot} on overall survival incidence, independent of treatment schedule, is shown in Fig. 3A. Patients with tumor T_{pot} values less than 4 days, i.e., relatively fast growing tumors, did significantly worse than patients with slower growing tumors (p = 0.02, log rank test). This indicates that T_{pot} has some prognostic significance. Correlation of T_{pot} with local control is shown in Fig. 3B, in which patients have been separated according to the radiotherapy schedule received, conventional (7.5 weeks) or accelerated (5 weeks). The most striking result is that the patients with fast-growing tumors (short pretreatment T_{pot}) treated with conventional radiotherapy had the worst local control.

Comments

These two randomized trials have already led to the following conclusions:

1. HF using two fractions per day has allowed the delivery of 80 Gy with better locoregional control than with 70 Gy using a single fraction per day, without increasing the incidence and severity of normal tissue damage.
2. The available results using three fractions of 1.6 Gy per day with 4-h intervals have demonstrated the feasibility of delivering 72 Gy in 45 fractions over 41/2–5 weeks. However, there is already a significant increase in acute morbidity and a trend towards an increase in severe late

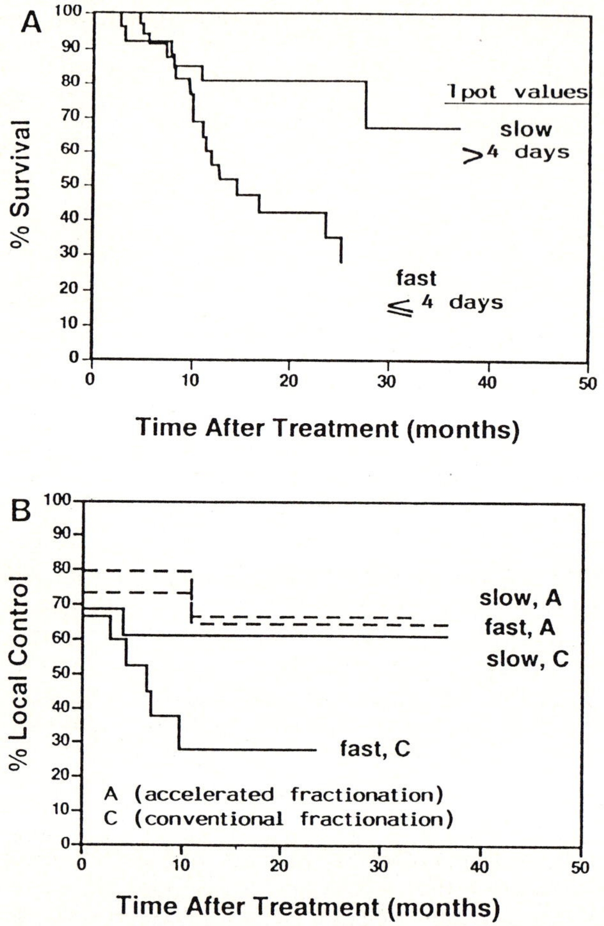

Fig. 3. A Actual survival of patients split according to the pretreatment T_{pot} (cell cycle time divided by the propostion of cells in cycle) values, independent of treatment arm. **B** Local control of tumors according to treatment arm and pretreatment T_{pot}

normal tissue injuries. These interim results suggest that this type of approach would only be of interest if a significant increase in locoregional control was achieved and/or if reliable criteria were available for the analysis of results; it seems that the correlation of T_{pot} values with locoregional control and survival provides these criteria. Improvement of this regime would require the extension of the interfraction time to 8 h in order to allow the maximum duration for the repair of sublethal damage in normal tissue. It seems difficult to further reduce the overall treatment time without decreasing the total dose below 70 Gy, and our experience with three AF trials and nearly 900 patients (Horiot et al. 1988a,b; Van den Bogaert et al. 1989) does not favour further reduction in dose and in overall treatment time.

Conclusions

An 11-year experience in the EORTC Cooperative Group of Radiotherapy with modified fractionation regimes allows a few firm conclusions to be drawn:

1. When exploring HF and AF, large randomized trials (300–500 patients) can only demonstrate significant variations in locoregional control.
2. Modern radiobiological data on repair of normal tissue damage and tumor repopulation constitute a reliable basis for the development of this type of trial and so far are highly consistent with the available results.
3. In head and neck cancers treated with curative intent, modified fractionation schemes seem to be the most promising approach to improve locoregional control.
4. Cell kinetics parameters should now be part of the data to be collected in all patients that enter fractionation trials. It is, however, premature to select patients for each type of radiotherapy scheme according to T_{pot} values or other predictive parameters.

References

Begg AC, McNally NJ, Shrieve DC et al. (1985) Method to measure the duration of DNA synthesis and the potential doubling time from a single sample. Cytometry 6:620–626

Begg AC, Hofland I, Moonen L et al. (1990) The predictive value of cell kinetic measurements in a European trial of accelerated fractionation in advanced head and neck tumors: an interim report. Int J Radiat Oncol Biol Phys 19:1449–1453

Horiot JC, Nabid A, Chaplain G et al. (1982) Clinical experience with multiple fractions per day (MFD) in the radiotherapy of head and neck carcinoma. J Eur Radiother 3(2):79–89

Horiot JC, van Den Bogaert W, Ang KK et al. (1988a) Trials using radiotherapy with multiple fractions per day. In: Banfi A, Lattvada A, Santoro A, Lucali R (eds) Radioterapia e trattamenti integrati. Casa Editrice Ambrosiana, Milan, pp 17–25

Horiot JC, van Den Bogaert W, Ang KK et al. (1988b) European Organization for Research on Treatment of Cancer trials using radiotherapy with multiple fractions per day. A 1978–1987 survey. In: Vaeth JM, Meyer J (eds) Frontiers of radiation therapy and oncology. Karger, Basel, pp 149–161

Van Den Bogaert W, Horiot JC, van der Schueren E (1989) Radiotherapy with multiple fractions per day. In: Steel GG, Adams GE, Horwich A (eds) The biological basis of radiotherapy, 2nd edn. Elsevier, Amsterdam, pp 209–222

Withers R, Horiot JC (1987) Hyperfractionation. In: Withers R, Peters LJ (eds) Innovations in radiation oncology. Springer, Berlin Heidelberg New York, pp 223–230

Second Primary Tumors in Oral and Oropharyngeal Cancer

N. de Vries

Department of Otolaryngology/Head and Neck Surgery, Free University Hospital, P.O. Box 7057, 1007MB, Amsterdam, the Netherlands

Introduction

Second primary tumors constitute a major problem in patients with squamous cell cancer of the head and neck. They occur in 15%–30% of cases, mainly in the upper aerodigestive tract (Gluckman et al. 1980; Hordijk and de Jong 1983; de Vries 1990). The majority of second primary tumors occur more than half a year after the index tumor and are called "metachronous"; when they occur within 6 months, they are called "synchronous." They occur more often in men than in women and usually have a bad prognosis, because they often occur at bad sites (lung/esophagus) or in already treated areas, rendering curative treatment difficult or impossible. In certain early stage diseases such as T1 N0 laryngeal cancer, the risk of death from a later lung cancer is greater than from the primary disease. For this reason, second primary tumors are regarded as the "overshadowing treat" for early stage head and neck cancer patients (Lippman and Hong 1989). Second tumors are one of the main reasons that despite many advances in the treatment of head and neck cancer (e.g., in reconstructive surgery or combined treatment modalities), long-term survival has only marginally increased in the past decades. Interest in the phenomenon has increased, and during the last 10 years, much has become known about their etiology, pathogenesis, frequency, and predilection sites. Research on the value of screening and (chemo)prevention has taken place and is still in progress. As well as having many similarities, there are important differences between the four sites of head and neck cancer: oral cavity, oropharynx, hypopharynx, and larynx, with regards to site relationships, frequency, and geographical and clinical differences. In laryngeal cancer, for example, many patients present with early stage disease and the 5-year survival rate is higher than 90%, making early detection or prevention measures more important than in oral, oro pharyngeal, and hypopharyngeal cancer, in which many patients present with advanced disease. In addition, predilection sites have been documented;

in laryngeal cancer, more than half of all second tumors occur in the lung, whereas in the three other sites, they occur spread over the whole upper aerodigestive tract. In this paper, we will focus exclusively on the problem of second tumors in oral and oropharyngeal cancer.

Etiology and Pathogenesis

The pathogenesis of oral and oropharyngeal cancer is multifactorially determined, and the same factors that caused the first tumor, such as tobacco and alcohol, also influence the development of a second tumor (Wynder et al. 1957, 1976, 1977; Williams and Horn 1977; Tuyns 1979; Rothman et al. 1980). In addition, genetic susceptility (de Vries et al. 1987; Schantz et al. 1990; Schantz and Hsu 1989; Spitz et al. 1989) plays a role.

Frequency of Multiple Primary Tumors in Oropharyngeal Cancer

The frequency of second tumors in oral and oropharyngeal cancer is comparable with that of hypopharyngeal cancer, but definitively higher than in laryngeal cancer. Few studies are devoted to second tumors of index tumors of these sites alone. In some studies, the oro- and hypopharynx or the naso-, oro-, and hypopharynx are taken together. The reported frequency of oral and oropharyngeal cancer is 7.1%–30.0% and 5.7%–28.4%, respectively (Tables 1 and 2). In one series on oral cancer, a division was made according to the location of the index tumor within the oral cavity (de Vries et al. 1986). The series showed that more second tumors occur in index tumors of the floor of mouth, inferior alveolar process, and retromolar trigone than in the rest of the oral cavity. No studies with actuarial survival rates or divisions according to site within the oropharynx have yet been carried out.

Management

As an adjunct to changes in life-style (cessation of smoking and drinking, dietary habits), two approaches will be discussed: early detection and (chemo-) prevention.

Early Detection

In many centers, panendoscopy is performed routinely during initial work-up (Atkins et al. 1984; McGuirt and Winston-Salem 1982; Leipzig 1983;

Table 1. Oral cancer: frequency, site, and time sequence of second primary tumors

Reference	Year	Total oral cancers reported (*n*)	SPT		UADT		Synchronous	Metachronous
			n	%	*n*	%	%	%
Berg et al.	1970	3443	248	7.1	110	3.2	–	–
Gluckman et al.	1980	158	28	17.7	24	15.1	–	–
Tepperman and Fitzpatrick	1981	337	101	30.0	82	24.3	–	–
Hordijk and de Jong	1983	152	26	17.1	22	14.4	–	–
Lamprecht et al.	1983	138	17	12.5	–	–	5.6	8.7
Black et al.	1983	1551	287	18.5	135	8.7	7.9	10.5
De Vries et al.	1985	210	38	18.0	23	11.0	1.9	16.1
Shikhani et al.	1986	437	57	13.0	46	10.5	6.1	6.9
Haughey et al.	1992	728	127	17.4	97	13.3	7.4	10.0

SPT, second primary tumor; UADT, upper aerodigestive tract.

Table 2. Oropharyngeal cancer: frequency, site, and time sequence of second primary tumors

Reference	Year	Total oral cancers reported (*n*)	SPT		UADT		Lung		Synchronous	Metachronous
			n	%	*n*	%	*n*	%	%	%
Healy et al.	1976	130	37	28.4	–	–	–	–	16.9	11.5
Gluckman et al.	1980	131	27	20.6	23	17.5	7	5.3	–	–
Hordijk and de Jong	1983	152	26	17.2	22	14.4	8	5.9	–	–
Lamprecht et al.	1983	156	9	5.7	–	–	–	–	2.5	3.2
Black et al.	1983	880	92	10.4	42	4.7	8	0.9	3.6	6.8
De Vries et al.	1985	113	17	15.0	10	9.3	–	–	2.6	12.4
Shikhani et al.	1986	339	45	13.6	36	10.9	15	4.5	6.4	7.2
Haughey et al.	1992	523	120	23	96	17	13	2.5	8.8	14.2

SPT, second primary tumor; UADT, upper aerodigestive tract.

Leipzig et al. 1985; Maisel and Vermeersch 1981; Schuller and Fritsch 1986; Neel 1984). Although in some studies a high frequency of synchronous tumors was found, meta-analysis has shown that only up to 2% were detected by panendoscopy alone, which implies that its cost-effectiveness has to be kept in mind constantly. It is rational to perform panendoscopy only in the highest risk groups, whereas it is irrational in elderly patients and in those with advanced disease, in poor general condition, or with large tumors with the risk of airway obstruction.

To complicate the problem, the majority of second tumors occur metachronously. Since biannual panendoscopy is unfeasible, restricting screening to lung cancer could be considered. The usual screening during follow-up is a once- or twice-yearly chest X-ray, but its value is questionable (Boysen et al. 1985; Engelen et al. 1993; Snow 1992; Lau et al. 1986; Wolfensberger 1988). Biannual bronchoscopy and sputum cytology is possibly more effective. In oral and oropharyngeal cancer, such studies have not yet been performed. However, data on laryngeal cancer can shed light on whether this kind of follow-up could be useful in oral and oropharyngeal cancer.

In a multicenter study in the Netherlands, the effectiveness of twice-yearly bronchoscopy as an adjunct to routine follow-up in patients with laryngeal cancer was investigated (Rachmat et al. 1992). In 170 selected patients, 500 bronchoscopies were performed. Five (2.8%) male patients developed lung cancer after a follow-up of 34 months. In only two of them was the diagnosis made by bronchoscopy. After treatment with curative intent, both developed a recurrent lung cancer. Rodriquez et al. (1984) performed twice-yearly bronchoscopy in 286 patients with laryngectomy for laryngeal cancer. In 36 patients (12.5%), a lung cancer was found during a follow-up of 3 years. In six of these 36 patients, the diagnosis of lung cancer was based on bronchoscopy alone.

In conclusion, the extra burden for patient and personnel and the cost-effectiveness does not justify routine bronchoscopy in the follow-up of laryngeal cancer. In oral and oropharyngeal cancer, the total frequency of second primary tumors is higher than in laryngeal cancer, but the percentage of secondaries in the lung is lower. Therefore, periodic bronchoscopy in these sites is unjustified as well.

Since screening in the follow-up is not useful in the total group of patients, it is to be investigated whether in the future a better identification of patients "at risk" may justify endoscopy in subgroups. Such risk factors could be based on gender, smoking and drinking habits, differences in human leukocyte antigens (HLA), immunoglobulin allotypes, vitamin A and beta-carotene serum levels, and DNA damage repair deficiencies (de Vries and Snow 1990; de Vries et al. 1987a,b; Schantz et al. 1990; Schantz and Hsu 1989; Spitz et al. 1989). Research into markers of mucosa at risk is also of importance (Copper et al. 1992).

Chemoprevention

Chemoprevention, defined as intervention in the process of carcinogenesis with dietary or chemical agents with the aim of preventing or delaying the development of cancer, offers an attractive alternative. Several clinical chemoprevention trials with beta-carotene, vitamin A, and other retinoids or with agents working alongside other mechanisms are at present being carried out (Table 3). Early stage head and neck cancer patients treated with curative intent form an ideal population on which to test chemopreventive medication because of the extremely high risk. Three studies will be discussed: in two of these, all sites within the head and neck were eligible, in one (EUROSCAN), only oral cavity and larynx.

M.D. Anderson Study

Hong et al. (1990) at the M.D. Anderson hospital published the results of the use of 50-100 mg 13-*cis* retinoic acid (isotretinoin) per square meter body surface area during 12 months in cured head and neck cancer patients. All stages and all the four sites (oral cavity, oropharynx, hypopharynx, and larynx) were eligible, In the 103 patients, only two (4%) second tumors occurred after a follow-up period of 32 months in the isotretinoin group ($n = 49$), as compared to 12 (24%) in the placebo group ($n = 51$). After 42 months, this frequency increased to three out of 49 (6%) versus 14 out of 51 (28%). These data showed for the first time that chemoprevention of second tumors in head and neck cancer is possible. However, the series was limited and the number of second tumors in the placebo group (24%) was exceptionally high (one would expect 5%–10% after 32 months), whereas the number of second tumors (4%) in the treated patients was exceptionally low. These encouraging data need to be confirmed by other studies. In addition, the toxicity of a dose of 50–100 mg 13-*cis* retinoic acid/m^2 was considerable. Hong and coworkers initiated a new trial in November 1991 with low-dose (30 mg) 13-*cis* retinoic acid, in which 1000 early stage patients will be included.

Groupe de Traitement des Tumeurs de la Tête et du Cou Study

In France, the Groupe de Traitement des Tumeurs de la Tête et du Cou (GETTEC) is performing a chemoprevention study in 323 patients (260 oral cavity and 62 oropharyngeal cancers), randomized between standard follow-up or follow-up and etrenitate (Tigason) at a dose of 50 mg in the first month and 25 mg in the following 23 months. Patients were entered from 1985 and entrance was stopped in December 1991.

Table 3. Chemoprevention trials in head and neck cancer

Institute	Years	Stage	Site	Drug/dose	*n*	Result
MD Anderson	1984–1990	All	All[a]	50–100 mg 13-*cis*-RA/m^2	103	+
GETTEC	1985–1991	Early	Oral cavity, oropharynx	50–25 mg Etrenitate	323	Awaited
EUROSCAN	1988–1993	Early	Oral cavity, larynx, lung	300 000 IU Retinol, 600 mg NAC	2400 of 2600 entered	Awaited
Connecticut	1990	Early	All[a]	50 mg Beta-carotene	600 planned	Awaited
MD Anderson	1991	Early	All[a]	30 mg 13-*cis* RA/m^2	1000 planned	Awaited
EUROSCAN II	1993	Early	All[a]	To be announced	4000 planned	

GETTEC, Groupe de Traitement des Tumeurs de la Tête et du Cou; RA, retinoic acid; NAC, *N*-acetyl-L-cysteine.
[a] All sites: oral cavity, oropharynx, hypopharynx, and larynx.

Euroscan

By far the largest chemoprevention study in early stage head and neck cancer is EUROSCAN (EUROSCAN Steering Committee 1990; de Vries et al. 1990, 1991), and this European study will be discussed in detail. EUROSCAN is an European Organization for Research on Treatment of Cancer (EORTC) chemoprevention study in patients with oral, laryngeal, and lung cancer treated with curative intent which started in June 1988. The chemopreventive drugs being used are 300 000 IU retinyl palmitate daily during 1 year and half this dose during a second year, or 600 mg *N*-acetyl-L-cysteine during 2 years, or both drugs, or neither, in a 2 × 2 factorial design (Stampfer et al. 1984). The rationable for the choice of these two drugs is discussed below.

Vitamin A. In vivo, in vitro, and in nutritional epidemiological studies, vitamin A and its precursor beta-carotene have been found to protect against epithelial cancer (Peto et al. 1981; Colditz et al. 1987; Byers 1988). A higher risk of lung cancer has been found in individuals with low intake and/or serum levels of retinol or beta-carotene (Ziegler et al. 1984; Byers et al. 1984; Menkes et al. 1986; Middleton et al. 1986). In several studies, low serum levels of vitamin A and/or beta-carotene correlated with head and neck squamous cell cancer and/or lung cancer (Bichler and Daxenbichler 1982; Fex et al. 1986; Friedman et al. 1986). Serum levels of vitamin A were shown to be lower in patients with head and neck cancer with second primary tumors ($n = 24$) than in those without ($n = 71$) (de Vries and Snow 1990).

Vitamin A has proven to be a relatively safe and nontoxic drug, even when given in high doses and for a long period (Silverman et al. 1963; Bendich and Langseth 1989). Retinyl palmitate (EUROSCAN) has been used for many years for skin diseases with acceptable side effects, and the dose of 300 000 IU daily is based on this experience. This dose causes justifiable side effects with response rates comparable to higher doses.

N-Acetyl-L-Cysteine. *N*-Acetyl-L-cysteine (NAC), a precursor of glutathione (Cotgreave et al. 1986), has attracted attention as a possible chemopreventive agent. It has potent antioxidant/detoxificant properties. In vitro, NAC inhibits mutagens such as aflatoxin, benzpyrene, and cigarette smoke condensate (de Flora et al. 1984, 1989; de Flora 1984). It prevents chemically induced lung and colon tumors in experimental animals. NAC added before and after the carcinogen exposure significantly reduced the incidence and multiplicity of lung tumors is mice and of colon tumors in the rat (de Flora et al. 1986; Wilpart et al. 1986). NAC is safe and without major side effects.

Vitamin A and N-Acetyl-L-Cysteine. NAC is thought to act in the early stages of carcinogenesis: before and possibly shortly after the occurrence of DNA damage; vitamin A, later: in the promotion and progression phases.

NAC as well as Vitamin A could be active as a single drug, while the combination theoretically cover almosts the whole carcinogenic process, whereas no interaction with regard to side effects is expected.

End Points and Accrual of EUROSCAN as of June 1, 1992. In total 2600 patients are planned. The end points of the EUROSCAN trial are second tumors, local/regional recurrence, and distant metastases as well as long-term survival rates. The study started on June 1, 1988. On October 1, 1993, 2400 of the 2600 patients planned had entered the study. On average, 40–50 new patients are entered per month. The accrual of the last 200 patients will end in 1993. A total of 63 cancer centers from 14 European countries are entering patients. Forty percent of the patients had lung cancer and 60% had head and neck cancer, 72% of which had laryngeal cancer.

Interim analysis of side effects and toxicity (de Vries et al. 1991) in 700 patients with sufficient follow-up as noted as of September 1, 1991, showed that the intervention is in general well tolerated and that the toxicity is mild.

Conclusion

In the management of second primary tumors in head and neck cancer, chemoprevention is more promising than intensified screening. It is gradually developing from an interesting experimental model to a realistic adjuvant treatment. The exciting data from Hong et al. (1990) need confirmation by larger studies using less toxic, but equally effective, drugs. In Europe, the EUROSCAN study is running successfully, and it might confirm that this experimental treatment is becoming a realistic form of intervention in cured head and neck cancer patients. When positive results are obtained in this and subsequent studies, chemopreventive agents in the future might be routinely applied in these extremely high-risk patients. The ideal drug or drug combination, the dose, and the duration have yet to be established.

References

Atkins JP, Keane WM, Young KA, Rowe LD (1984) Value of panendoscopy in determination of second primary cancer. A study of 451 cases of head and neck cancer. Arch Otolaryngol 110:533–534

Bendich L, Langseth H (1989) Safety of vitamin A. Am J Clin Nutr 49:358–371

Berg JW, Schottenfeld D, Ritter F (1970) Incidence of multiple primary cancer: 3. Cancers of the respiratory and upper digestive system as multiple primary cancers. J Natl Cancer Inst 44:263–274

Bichler E, Daxenbichler G (1982) Retinoic acid-binding protein in human squamous cell carcinomas of the ORL region. Cancer 49:619–621

Black RJ, Gluckman JL, Shumrick DA (1983) Multiple primary tumors of the upper aerodigestive tract. Clin Otolaryngol 8:277–281

Boysen M, Natvig K, Winther FO, Tausjo J (1985) Value of routine follow-up in patients treated for squamous cell carcinoma of the head and neck. J Otolaryngol 14:211–217

Byers T (1988) Diet and cancer: any progress in the interim? Cancer 62:1713–1724

Byers T, Vena J, Mettlin C, Swansons M, Graham S (1984) Dietary vitamin A and lung cancer risk: an analysis by histologic subtypes. Am J Epidemiol 120:769–776

Colditz GA, Stampfer MJ, Willett WC (1987) Diet and lung cancer: a review of the epidemiologic evidence in humans. Arch Intern Med 147:157–160

Copper MP, Braakhuis BJM, Vries N de, Dongen van GAMS, Nauta JP, Snow GB (1993) A panel of biomarkers of carcinogenesis of the upper aerodigestive tract as potential intermediate endpoints in chemoprevention trials. Cancer 71:825–890

Cotgreave IA, Grafstrom RC, Moldeus P (1986) Modulation of pneumotoxicity by cellular glutathione and precursors. Bull Eur Physiolpathol Respir [Suppl] 22:2635–2665

De Flora S (1984) Detoxification of genotoxic compounds as a threshold mechanism limiting their carcinogenicity. Toxicol Pathol 12:337–343

De Flora S, Bennicelli C, Zanacchi P et al. (1984) In vitro effects of N-acetylcysteine on the mutagenicity of direct acting compounds and procarcinogens. Carcinogenesis 5:505–510

De Flora S, Astengo M, Serra D, Benicelli C (1986) Prevention of induced lung tumours in mice by dietary N-acetylcysteine. Cancer Lett 32:235–241

De Flora S, Benicelli C, Caimalano R (1989) Inhibition of mutagenesis with N-acetylcysteine (NAC). In: Cerutti PA (ed) Anticarcinogenesis and radiation protection, p 373. Plenum, Milano

De Vries N (1990) The magnitude of the problem. In: de Vries N, Gluckman JL (eds) Multiple primary tumors in the head and neck, Thieme, Stuttgart, pp 1–29

De Vries N, Snow GB (1990) Relationship of vitamins A and E and beta-carotene serum levels to head and neck cancer patients with and without second primary tumors. Eur Arch ORL 247:368–370

De Vries N, Waal I van der, Snow GB (1985) Dubbeltumoren bij patienten met een plaveiselcelcarcinoom van het slijmvlies in het hoofdhalsgebied. Ned Tijdschr Geneeskd 129:1734–1738

De Vries N, de Lange G, Drexhage HA, Snow GB (1987a) Immunoglobulin allotypes in head and neck cancer patients with multiple primary tumors. Acta Otolaryngol 104:187–191

De Vries N, de Waal LP, de Lange G, Drexhage HA, Snow GB (1987b) HLA antigens and immunoglobulin allotypes in head and neck cancer patients with and without multiple primary tumors. Cancer 60:957–961

De Vries N, Zandwijk N van Pastorino U, McVie JC, Dalesio O, Snow GB (1990) Euroscan. Eur Cancer News 3:1–3

De Vries N, van Zandwijk N, Pastorino U (1991) The Euroscan study (guest editorial). Br J Cancer 64:985–989

Engelen AM, Stalpers LJA, Manni JJ, Ruijs JHJ, van Daal WAJ (1992) Yearly chest radiography in the early detection of lung cancer following laryngeal cancer (in press)

EUROSCAN Steering Committee (1990) Euroscan: EORTC study on screening and chemoprevention with vitamin A and/or N-acetyl-cysteine. Eur Cancer News 3:12–14

Fex G, Wahlberg P, Biorklund A, Wennerberg J, Willen R (1986) Studies of cellular retinol-binding protein (CRBP) in squamous-cell carcinomas of the head and neck region. Int J Cancer 37:217–221

Friedman GD, Blaner WS, Goodman DS et al. (1986) Serum retinol and retinol-binding protein levels do not predict subsequent lung cancer. Am J Epidemiol 123:781–789

Gluckman JL, Crissman JD, Donegan JO (1980) Multicentric squamous cell carcinoma of the upper aerodigestive tract. Head Neck Surg 3:90–96
Haughey BH, Gates GA, Arfken CL, Harvey J (1992) Meta-analysis of second malignant tumors in head and neck cancer: the case for an endoscopic screening protocol. Ann Otol Rhinol Laryngol 101:105–112
Healy GB, Strong MS, Uchmakli A, Vaughan CW, DiTroia JF (1976) Carcinoma of the palatine arch. Am J Surg 131:498–503
Heeringa A, de Vries N, Snow GB, Stam J (1988) Laryngeal cancer and lung cancer in the same patient: a retrospective study. Eur J Surg Oncol 14:209–211
Hong WK, Lippman SM, Itri LM et al. (1990) Prevention of second tumors with isotretinoin in squamous-cell carcinoma of the head and neck. N Engl J Med 323:795–798
Hordijk GJ, de Jong JMA (1983) Synchronous and metachronous tumours in patients with head and neck cancer. J Laryngol Otol 97:619–621
Lamprecht J, Lamprecht A, Morgenstern C (1983) Mehrfachtumoren im oberen Aerodigestivtract – eine retrospective Studies. Laryngol Rhinol Otol 62:499–501
Lau WF, Siu KF, Wei W, Lam KH (1986) Prospective screening for multiple tumors of the upper aerodigestive tract: a simple routine procedure. Laryngoscope 96:1149–1153
Leipzig B (1983) Bronchoscopy in the staging and evaluation of head and neck carcinoma. Ann Otol Rhinol Laryngol 92:373–376
Leipzig B, Zellmer JE, Klug D (1985) The role of endoscopy in evaluating patient with head and neck cancer. A multi-institutional prospective study. Arch Otolaryngol 111:589–593
Lippman SM, Hong WK (1989) Second malignant tumors in head and neck squamous cell carcinoma: the overshadowing threat for patients with early stage disease. Int J Radiat Oncol Biol Phys 17:691–695
Maisel RH, Vermeersch H (1981) Panendoscopy for second primaries in head and neck cancer. Ann Otol 90:460–464
McGuirt WF, Winston-Salem NC (1982) Panendoscopy as a screening examination for simultaneous primary tumors in head and neck cancer: a prospective sequential study and review of the literature. Laryngoscope 92:569–576
Menkes MS, Comstock GW, Vuilleumier JP, Helsing KJ, Ruder AA, Brook-meyer R (1986) Serum beta-carotene, vitamins A and E, selenium, and the risk of lung cancer. N Engl J Med 315:1250–1254
Middleton B, Byers T, Marshall J, Graham S (1986) Dietary vitamin A and cancer. Nutr Cancer 8:107–116
Neel HB (1984) Routine panendoscopy – is it necessary every time? Arch Otolaryngol 110:531–532
Peto R, Doll R, Buckley JD, Sporn MB (1981) Can dietary beta-carotene materially reduce human cancer rates? Nature 290:201–208
Rachmat L, Vreeburg G, de Vries N, Lubsen H, Hordijk GJ, van den Broek P, Snow GB (1993) The value of twice yearly bronchoscopy in the follow-up of patients with laryngeal cancer. Eur J Cancer 29a:1096–1099
Rodrìquez E, Castella J, Andrés L de, Cornudella R (1984) Lung cancer in patients with tracheostomy due to cancer of the larynx. Respiration 46:323–327
Rothman K, Cann CI, Flanders D, Fried MP (1980) Epidemiology of laryngeal cancer. Epidemiol Rev 2:196–213
Schantz SP, Hsu TC (1989) Mutagen-induced chromosome fragility within peripheral blood lymphocytes of head and neck cancer patients. Head Neck Surg 11: 337–341
Schantz SP, Spitz MR, Hsu TC (1990) Mutagen sensitivity in patients with head and neck cancers: a biological marker for risk of multiple primary malignancies. J Natl Cancer Inst 82:1773–1776

Schuller DE, Fritsch MH (1986) An assessment of the value of triple endoscopy in the evaluation of head and neck cancer patients. J Surg Oncol 32:156–158

Shikhani AH, Matanoski GM, Jones MM, Koshina HK, Johns ME (1986) Multiple pri-mary malignancies in head and neck cancer patients. Arch Otolaryngol 112:1172–1180

Silverman S, Renstrup G, Pindborg J (1963) Studies in oral leukoplakias: III. Effects of vitamin A comparing clinical, histopathological, cytologic and hematologic responses. Acta Odontol Scand 21:271–279

Snow GB (1992) Follow-up in head and neck cancer (guest editorial). Eur J Cancer 28:315–316

Spitz MR, Fueger JJ, Beddingfield NA et al. (1989) Chromosome sensitivity to bleomycin-induced mutagenesis, an independent risk factor for upper aerodigestive tract cancers. Cancer Res 49:4626–4650

Stampfer MJ, Buring JE, Willett W, Rosner B, Eberlein K, Hennekens CH (1984) The 2 × 2 factorial design: its application to a randomized trial of aspirin and carotene in U.S. physicians. Stat Med 4:111–116

Tepperman BS, Fitzpatrick PJ (1981) Second respiratory and upper digestive tract cancers after oral cancer. Lancet ii:547–549

Tuyns AJ (1979) Epidemiology of alcohol and cancer. Cancer Res 39:2840–2851

Williams RR, Horn JW (1977) Association of cancer sites with tobacco and alcohol consumption and socioeconomic status of patients: interview study from the third national cancer survey. J Netl Cancer Inst 58:525–547

Wilpart M, Speder D, Robertfroid M (1986) Anti-initiation activity of N-acetylcysteine in experimental colonic carcinogenesis. Cancer Lett 31:319–324

Wolfensberger M (1988) Aufwand und Nutzen regelmäßiger Nachkontrollen bei Patienten mit Pflasterzellkarzinomen des Larynx, der Mundhöhle und des Pharynx. HNO 36:28–32

Wynder EL, Bross ID, Feldman RM (1957) A study of etiological factors in cancer of the mouth. Cancer 10:1300–1323

Wynder EL, Covey LS, Mabuchi H (1976) Environmental factors in cancer of the larynx. Cancer 38:1591–1601

Wynder EL, Mushinski MH, Spivak JC (1977) Tobacco and alcohol consumption in relation to the development of multiple primary cancers. Cancer 40:1872–1878

Ziegler RG, Mason TJ, Stemhagen N et al. (1984) Dietary carotene and vitamin A and risk of lung cancer among white men in New Jersey. J Natl Cancer Inst 73:1429–1435

Induction Chemotherapy for Organ Preservation in Advanced Squamous Cell Carcinoma of the Oral Cavity and Oropharynx

G.T. Wolf[1], S. Urba[2], and M. Hazuka[3]

[1] Department of Otolaryngology – Head and Neck Surgery, University of Michigan Medical Center, Ann Arbor, MI 48109, USA
[2] Department of Internal Medicine, University of Michigan Medical Center, Ann Arbor, MI 48109, USA
[3] Department of Radiation Oncology, University of Michigan Medical Center, Ann Arbor, MI 48109, USA

Introduction

Squamous carcinoma of the upper aerodigestive tract comprises 5% of new cancer cases each year and accounts for 12000–15000 deaths. It is estimated that over 30000 new cases of oral cavity and pharynx cancer occur each year (Silverberg et al. 1990). Two thirds of these will be advanced (stage III or IV) at time of diagnosis. Conventional treatment strategies for these patients consist of combinations of radical surgical resection and postoperative radiation therapy and are associated with dismal 3-year survival rates ranging from 0%–50%. Furthermore, these treatment approaches result in significant functional and cosmetic disabilities due to radical resections of the tongue, mandible, pharynx, and larynx. Despite continuing refinements in surgical reconstruction, cancers arising in the oral cavity and pharynx consistently result in significant impairments in speech and swallowing that seriously affect quality of life.

In the early 1970s, preoperative or induction chemotherapy was introduced into the management of patients with locally advanced head and neck squamous cell carcinoma (Tarpley et al. 1975). With it, a new frontier in head and neck oncology was opened for exploration. The ensuing two decades saw the completion of a large number of randomized clinical trials designed to determine whether the addition of induction chemotherapy to conventional treatment enhanced survival rates in patients with stage III and IV cancers (Table 1). These experiences demonstrated the feasibility of induction chemotherapy and solidified a new multidisciplinary approach to head and neck cancers which included medical oncology, radiation oncology, and surgery. Unfortunately, despite these positive developments, the results of randomized trials failed to document a significant survival benefit from the addition of induction chemotherapy.

A secondary goal of these early studies was to develop preoperative drug regimens that could be effective enough to allow reductions in the

Table 1. Randomized trials of induction chemotherapy

Author	Patients	Chemotherapy	CR rate (%)	Results
Head and Neck Contracts Program (1987)	443	DDP+BLM	3	No difference in 5-year survival rate
Taylor et al. (1985)	95	MTX	6	No difference in 3-year survival rate
Toohill et al. (1987)	60	DDP+5-FU	18	Improved survival – standard therapy arm
Schuller et al. (1988)	158	DDP, BLM, MTX VCR	19	No survival difference
Martin et al. (1990)	75	DDP, 5-FU	46	No difference in 1-year survival rate
Holoye et al. (1985)	83	BLM, CTX, MTX 5-FU	5	No difference in 2-year survival rate

HNCP, Head and Neck Contracts Program; CR, complete rate; DDP, cisplatin; 5-FU, 5-fluorouracil; CTX, cytoxin; BLM, bleomycin; VCR, vincristine; MTX, methotrexate.

magnitude of radical surgical resection and reduce the functional and cosmetic morbidity of treatment. Although this goal was not achieved, results of prospective studies did provide important new observations which led to new strategies of organ-sparing treatment approaches for patients with oral cavity and oropharyngeal cancers. These initial studies demonstrated that several cycles of intensive induction chemotherapy were feasible and well tolerated and were associated with clinically complete tumor regressions in 30%–50% of previously untreated patients (Table 2). Clinically complete tumor regressions after induction chemotherapy were associated with prolonged survival compared to nonresponders (Kies et al. 1985; Al-Kourainy et al. 1987; Ervin et al. 1987). Finally, the response to induction chemotherapy seemed to predict success of subsequent radiation therapy (Ensley et al. 1984; Hong et al. 1985). These various observations, taken together, suggested to investigators that if prognostically favorable patients were identified by their tumor response to chemotherapy and if tumor extent could be reduced to a microscopic amount, then tumor cure might be achieved with definitive radiation therapy alone. Surgery could be held in reserve for salvage of persistent or recurrent cancer or for early treatment of chemotherapy nonresponders. Such an approach would have significant benefit, particularly for patients with large cancers of the tongue or pharynx, where radical excisions are associated with serious speech and swallowing morbidity, or patients with posterior tongue resections, which often necessitate concomitant laryngectomy.

Early Studies

Initial experiences with induction chemotherapy consisted of intermediate-dose methotrexate prior to surgery (Tarpley et al. 1975). Others utilized very high doses of methotrexate with leucovorin rescue (Ervin et al. 1981). Both demonstrated the feasibility of intensive drug administration prior to surgery. With the introduction of cisplatin, combination drug regimens incorporating this new, highly active agent with other active drugs such as bleomycin and methotrexate were developed in anticipation of response rates higher than single agent regimens. The earliest large randomized study of induction chemotherapy was initiated in 1980 by the National Cancer Institute in the United States and used cisplatin and bleomycin administered as a single course prior to surgery and radiation therapy (Head and Neck Contracts Program 1987). This treatment was compared to conventional surgery and radiation or to induction chemotherapy, surgery, and radiation followed by 6 months of monthly maintenance chemotherapy using cisplatin alone. Although no significant improvement in overall survival was achieved, the combination of induction and maintenance chemotherapy treatment did demonstrate a significant delay in the development of distant metastases. However, delivery of maintenance chemotherapy was difficult,

Table 2. Induction chemotherapy trials with platinum and fluorouracil

Investigator	Chemotherapy	Cycles	Evaluable patients	Response rate (%)	Complete response rate (%)
Kish et al. (1982)	Cisplatin (100 mg/m^2) 5-FU (1 gm/m^2 × 4 days)	2	26	88	20
Weaver et al. (1982)	Cisplatin (100 mg/m^2) 5-FU (1 gm/m^2 × 5 days)	3	88	93	54
Vokes et al. (1990)	Cisplatin (100 mg/m^2) 5-FU (1 gm/m^2 × 5 days) Leucovorin (100 mg/m^2 q4h × 5 days)	2	29	90	31
Kish et al. (1989)	Carboplatin (360 mg/m^2) 5-FU (1 gm/m^2 × 5 days) q28d	2–3	23[a]	59	18
Volling et al. (1989)	Carboplatin (300 mg/m^2) 5-FU (1 gm/m^2 × 5 days) q28d	3	52	87	33
Urba et al. (1992)	Carboplatin (400 mg/m^2) 5-FU (1 gm/m^2 × 5 days) q21d	3	44	89	50[b]

[a] Stage IV patients only.
[b] Primary tumor response.

and only one third of patients completed three cycles of the maintenance therapy. During this same period, Al-Sarraf and colleagues (Weaver et al. 1982) developed an induction regimen consisting of cisplatin and 5-fluorouracil (5-FU) as an alternative to bleomycin for patients with poor pulmonary function. This regimen proved to be highly active with complete response rates in the range of 30%–50% (Decker et al. 1983; Table 2). These and other investigators noted that some patients refused surgery after achieving a complete response to chemotherapy (Weaver et al. 1982). Many of these patients were treated with radiation therapy as an alternative and achieved long-term disease control. When survival rates of treated patients were analyzed according to response to induction chemotherapy, investigators consistently demonstrated that achievement of a response to chemotherapy was associated with prolonged survival (Wolf 1984). Not only did response predict favorable prognosis, but response appeared to predict subsequent radiation sensitivity of the cancer. These various observations lent support to the concept that definitive radiation therapy after achievement of a complete response to induction chemotherapy could be a highly effective treatment strategy that might maximize preservation of organ structure and function (Hong et al. 1985).

Pilot Studies of Organ Preservation

Jacobs et al. (1987) and Hong et al. (1985) were the first investigators to describe treatment approaches using chemotherapy and radiation with surgery held in reserve for salvage. Jacobs treated 30 patients with three cycles of cisplatin and 5-FU. Thirteen achieved a complete response and therefore were treated with full course radiation therapy. All patients who did not achieve a complete histologic response at the primary tumor site underwent definitive surgery and radiation. Overall 5-year survival for the entire group was reported as 44% (median follow-up 75 months). The overall survival for the patients achieving a complete response and organ preservation was 59%. These long-term results demonstrated the durability of this treatment approach for tumor control and suggested that organ preservation could be achieved in select patients. Similar long-term results have been reported by Hong's group (Karp et al. 1988). These early investigations included patients with squamous carcinomas arising from a variety of sites in the head and neck, including the oral cavity and oropharynx.

Induction Chemotherapy for Organ Preservation in Cancer of the Larynx

The only completed prospective randomized trial of induction chemotherapy combined with radiation and surgery salvage with the intent of organ preservation was conducted by the U.S. Department of Veterans' Affairs in patients with stage III and IV laryngeal cancer (Department of Veterans' Affairs Laryngeal Cancer Study Group 1991). A total of 332 patients were randomly and equally assigned to either three cycles of cisplatin (100 mg/m^2, day 1) and 5-FU (1000 mg/m^2 daily for 5 days) and radiation therapy or conventional surgery and radiation therapy. Patients randomized to the experimental treatment who did not achieve at least a 50% reduction in primary tumor size after two cycles of induction chemotherapy underwent immediate planned salvage surgery and postoperative radiation. With a median follow-up of 33 months, overall and disease-free survival rates were similar in the two treatment groups. Estimated 2-year survival was 68%. A total of 64% of patients randomized to induction chemotherapy were able to avoid laryngectomy. These results were viewed as very encouraging, since the patients treated were not highly selected and had very advanced laryngeal cancer. Nearly 25% required pretreatment tracheostomy because of airway obstruction, and half had clinically evident regional metastases. The results reported by the Veterans' Affairs Laryngeal Cancer Study Group were similar to the survival and organ preservation rates reported with radiation alone in smaller retrospective studies consisting of highly selected patients having primarily T3 or early T4 lesions and no neck nodes (Croll et al. 1989; Harwood et al. 1980, 1982). When nodal disease was present, however, 5-year survival rates with radiation alone were decreased from 50% to less than 25% (Harwood et al. 1983).

Although the results achieved with organ preservation in laryngeal cancer cannot be directly extrapolated to patients with cancers of the oral cavity, the pilot data and the randomized data were clearly encouraging enough to warrant further investigations in patients with cancers of other sites. Some of the early experiences and observations learned from the laryngeal preservation treatment approach, however, could be directly applied to other cancer sites. In particular, the Veterans' Affairs larynx study provided important information regarding the effectiveness of this organ-preserving treatment approach for managing regional metastases. A subset analysis of 92 patients with N2 or N3 neck disease was performed to determine the effectiveness of induction chemotherapy and radiation in patients with advanced regional metastases (Wolf and Fisher 1992). A total of 46 such patients were allocated to each treatment arm. Although there were no differences in overall survival between treatment arms for this subgroup, the patients achieving a complete response of the neck nodes showed improved survival compared to the surgery group. For those patients with less than a complete response in the neck, the overall death rate was significantly increased and survival time was decreased. These findings were primarily related to failure to control the disease in the neck even with salvage neck dissection. The results suggested that delay in detection of recurrent neck disease may have been important, since neck disease was often discovered to be unresectable at time of salvage neck dissection. Similar results indicating poor regional control of disease in the absence of a complete response after induction therapy were reported by Clark et al. (1991).

Complication rates after chemotherapy and radiation for organ preservation may be increased when salvage surgery is necessary. Although no increase in frequency or severity of surgical complications was seen with salvage surgery performed after a failure of induction chemotherapy, increases in the severity of surgical complications were found after salvage procedures performed after chemotherapy and radiation.

These various observations have prompted modifications in the surgical component of second generation organ preservation treatment protocols. We now perform planned neck dissections after chemotherapy for patients whose neck nodes have not shown complete regression. Neck dissection therefore precedes definitive radiation to the primary site and neck. Although this is a departure from traditional surgical oncologic principles, pilot data supports the feasibility of this approach, particularly if radiation therapy is not delayed more than 2 weeks after neck dissection (Byers et al. 1991). Further, special care is taken in salvaging chemoradiation failures, including meticulous attention to nutrition, tissue handling, thyroid status, electrolyte balance, and liberal use of vascularized flap reconstructions and control fistulae.

Induction Chemotherapy for Organ Preservation in Cancer of the Oral Cavity and Oropharynx

In 1986, an aggressive induction chemotherapy protocol for organ preservation in patients with advanced cancers of the oral cavity/oropharynx was initiated at the University of Michigan (Urba et al. 1989). Patients were treated with mitoguazone (400–500 mg/m^2 on days 1 and 8), cisplatin (30 mg/m^2 per day, continuous infusion days 8–12), and 5-FU (1000 mg/m^2 per day, continuous infusion days 8–12). Mitoguazone was used in an attempt to synchronize tumor cells in S or G2 phase. Three cycles of chemotherapy were administered at 28-day intervals as induction therapy. Patients with tumors downstaged to at least T1 or N1 size after chemotherapy were eligible to receive definitive radiation therapy. All others underwent salvage surgery. Although the overall response rate to the induction regimen was quite high (46% complete response), toxicity was appreciable, with two deaths attributed to drug treatment. Over 80% of the clinical complete response patients who underwent biopsy were also histologically negative. Of 33 patients, six had oral cavity carcinoma and 27 had oropharynx carcinoma. Organ preservation was achieved in two of six oral cavity patients (33%) and 16 of 27 oropharynx patients (59%). Although the organ preservation rates were not as high as in patients with laryngeal cancer, overall survival rates with this regimen were similar to a historical control group of 152 patients treated with conventional surgery and radiation for similar stage III or IV tumors. This study was completed before difficulties in control of advanced neck disease were realized and before the severity of complications with salvage surgery were fully appreciated.

In our more recent study for patients with advanced nonlaryngeal cancers (Urba et al. 1992), carboplatin and 5-FU are used as induction therapy, and neck dissection is included prior to radiation for patients who do not achieve a complete response in the neck nodes. Of 26 oral cavity/oropharynx patients treated thus far, 62% achieved a complete response at the primary site. Organ preservation has been achieved in 19 of 26 patients (73%). With short follow-up (less than 2 years), 92% of patients are alive without evidence of disease.

Other investigators have begun reporting similar results. Pfister et al. (1992) treated 33 patients with advanced resectable cancer of the tongue base or tonsil with one to three cycles of cisplatin-based induction chemotherapy. Patients with less than a partial response had standard surgery and postoperative radiation. Patients with greater than a partial response of the primary tumor received definitive radiation. With a median follow-up of 31 months, they reported a 2-year survival rate of 56% and estimated a 5-year survival rate of 42%. Preservation of the larynx was achieved in 54% of patients and tongue preservation in 76%.

Significant Unanswered Questions

Significant questions remain as to the role of induction chemotherapy for organ preservation in patients with head and neck cancer. What is the real benefit and does induction chemotherapy enhance the effectiveness of radiation therapy? One thing that is clear is that overall survival rates have not been changed. Therefore, are the additional costs, length of treatment, and morbidity associated with induction chemotherapy justified, particularly when as many as 50% of the treated patients may also eventually require salvage surgery? These remain unanswered questions at the present time. Further organ preservation trials must address quality of life issues and carefully analyze true differences in functional capabilities. For laryngeal cancer patients, the value of preservation of the larynx is intuitively obvious. For oral cavity and oropharynx patients, wherever improving surgical reconstructions are possible, the advantages may be less obvious. Studies of oral function after successful chemoradiation have not been reported, and there have been no direct comparisons to modern surgical resection and reconstruction. Further, the oncologic safety of organ preservation for specific situations is unknown, such as when tumor invades the mandible or when direct tumor extension to the soft tissue of the neck is present. In such situations, radiation alone is not exceptionally effective, and the addition of chemotherapy may not be efficacious enough to achieve results comparable to surgical resection.

In conjunction with these unknown factors, the complication rates following salvage surgery must be considered. The ability of patients to return to usual social activities, regular diet, and even full employment must also be measured. How are the economics of such preserved or restored function measured against the economics of treatment costs? Clearly, our preliminary experiences have suggested that for the individual with successful organ preservation, the economic cost is well justified.

Is induction chemotherapy beneficial in terms of overall control? Although overwhelming evidence suggests that survival is not enhanced when induction chemotherapy is added to surgery, the results in advanced laryngeal cancer do suggest that the chemotherapy may be additive to radiation in overall cancer control for some patients with very advanced disease. It remains unclear whether induction chemotherapy can have a beneficial effect on systemic metastases. Several studies have suggested improved rates of distant metastases (Head and Neck Contracts Program 1987; Schuller et al. 1988; Al-Sarraf et al. 1992), but the data are difficult to interpret, since in most cases the improvement in distant metastases is reported as an analysis of site of first failure rather than overall rate of failure.

The appropriate goal in future trials must be improved survival. For advanced disease patients this most likely will require continued exploration of more aggressive local therapy combined with systemic adjuvant chemotherapy or immunotherapy directed at disseminated disease.

It is important to not lose sight of the fact that the success of these innovative organ preservation treatment approaches has been predicated in the use of initial chemotherapy to select patients having a favorable prognosis and the planned integration of early salvage surgery. Intensive work is underway in conjunction with the current induction chemotherapy studies to try and identify those biologic and tumor characteristics that are predictive of both tumor behavior and response to therapy. With such tools, individual selection of patients for specific therapy and more precise refinement in therapies will be possible to achieve maximal organ preservation with minimal treatment morbidity.

Continued clinical trial research is clearly indicated. Such studies must be carefully designed to maximize patient safety and must ensure close collaboration and cooperation among the various investigators representing the fields of surgery, medical oncology, and radiation oncology. Experimental treatment outside of the clinical trial setting is not to be condoned. As further experience is gained and other randomized trials are completed, it is hoped that organ preservation approaches may become accepted alternatives to radical surgical extirpations for patients with advanced cancers of the oral cavity and oropharynx.

References

Al-Kourainy K, Kish J, Ensley J et al. (1987) Achievement of superior survival for histologically negative versus histologically positive complete responders to cisplatin combination in patients with locally advanced head and neck cancer. Cancer 99:233–238

Al-Sarraf M, Scott CB, Ahmad K et al. (1992) Phase III study comparing sequential chemotherapy and radiotherapy to radiotherapy for resected and negative margins in squamous cell carcinoma of the head and neck: intergoup study #0034. Proc Am Soc Clin Oncol 11:242

Byers RM, Clagman GL, Guillainodegui OM et al. (1991) Resection of advanced cervical metastasis prior to definitive radiotherapy for primary squamous carcinomas of the upper aerodigestive tract. 37th annual proceedings of the Society for Head Neck Surgery, Maui, p 68

Clark J, Busse P, Norris C et al. (1991) Regional control after induction therapy for head and neck cancer: an analysis of 303 patients and a proposal for management of the neck. Proc Am Soc Clin Oncol 10:197

Croll GA, Gerritson GJ, Tiwari RS et al. (1989) Primary radiotherapy with surgery in reserve for advanced laryngeal carcinoma: results and complications. Eur J Surg Oncol 15:350–356

Decker DA, Drelichman A, Jacobs J et al. (1983) Adjuvant chemotherapy for advanced head and neck squamous carcinoma. Cancer 60:301–311

Department of Veterans' Affairs Laryngeal Cancer Study Group (1991) Induction chemotherapy plus radiation compared with surgery plus radiation in patients with advanced laryngeal cancer. N Engl J Med 324:1685–1690

Ensley JF, Jacobs JR, Weaver A et al. (1984) Correlation between response to cisplatin-combination chemotherapy and subsequent radiotherapy in previously untreated patients with advanced squamous cell cancers of the head and neck. Cancer 54:811–814

Ervin TJ, Kirkwood J, Weichiselbaum RR et al. (1981) Improved survival for patients with advanced carcinoma of the head and neck treated with methotrexate–leucovorin prior to definitive radiotherapy or surgery. Laryngoscope 91:1181–1190

Ervin TS, Clark JR, Weichselbaum RR et al. (1987) An analysis of induction and adjuvant chemotherapy in the multidisciplinary treatment of squamous cell carcinoma of the head and neck. J Clin Oncol 5:10–20

Harwood AR, Bryce DP, Rider WO (1980) Management of T_3 glottic cancer. Arch Otolaryngol 106:697–699

Harwood AR, ENT Group (1982) The management of advanced supraglottic carcinoma by delayed combined therapy. Int J Radiat Oncol Biol Phys 8:101–102

Harwood AR, Bealer FA, Cummings BJ (1983) Supraglottic laryngeal carcinoma: an analysis of dose–time–volume factors in 410 patients. Int J Radiat Oncol Biol Phys 9:311–319

Head and Neck Contracts Program (1987) Adjuvant chemotherapy for advanced head and neck squamous carcinoma. Cancer 60:301–311

Holoye PY, Grossman TW, Toohill RJ et al. (1985) Randomized study of adjuvant chemotherapy for head and neck cancer. Otolaryngol Head Neck Surg 93:712–715

Hong WK, O'Donoghue GM, Sheetz S et al. (1985) Sequential response patterns to chemotherapy and radiotherapy in head and neck cancer: potential impact to treatment in advanced laryngeal cancer. Prog Oncol Res 201:191–197

Jacobs C, Goffinet DR, Goffinet L et al. (1987) Chemotherapy as a substitute for surgery in the treatment of advanced resectable head and neck cancer. Cancer 60:1178–1183

Karp D, Carter R, Vaugh C et al. (1988) Voice preservation using induction chemotherapy plus radiation therapy as an alternative to laryngectomy in advanced head and neck cancer long term follow-up. Proc Am Soc Clin Oncol 7:152
Kies MS, Gordan LI, Hauck WW et al. (1985) Analysis of complete responders after initial treatment with chemotherapy in head and neck cancer. Otolaryngol Head Neck Surg 93:199–205
Kish J, Drechman A, Peppard S et al. (1982) Clinical trial of cisplatin and 5-fluorouracil as initial treatment of advanced squamous cell carcinoma of the head and neck. Cancer Treat Rep 66:471–474
Kish J, Ensley JF, Tapazoglou E, Al-Saraf M (1989) Carboplatin and 5-FU infusion as an effective outpatient induction chemotherapy in patients with locally advanced head and neck cancer. Proc Am Soc Clin Oncol 8:173
Martin M, Hazan A, Vergnes L et al. (1990) Randomized study of 5-fluorouracil and cisplatin as neoadjuvant therapy in head and neck cancer: a preliminary report. Int J Radiat Oncol Biol Phys 19:973–975
Pfister DG, Harrison L, Strong EW et al. (1992) Organ/function preservation in advanced oropharynx cancer: results with induction chemotherapy and radiation. Proc Am Soc Clin Oncol 11:241
Pinto HA, Jacobs C, van Der Pas M et al. (1991) Long-term follow-up of organ preservation in advanced resectable head and neck cancer. Proc Am Soc Clin Oncol 10:207
Schuller DE, Metch B, Stein DW et al. (1988) Preoperative chemotherapy in advanced resectable head and neck cancer: final report of the southwest oncology group. Laryngoscope 98:1205–1211
Silverberg E, Boray CC, Squires TS (1990) Cancer statistics. Cancer 40:9–26
Tarpley JL, Chretien PB, Alexander JC et al. (1975) High dose methotrexate as a preoperative adjuvant in the treatment of epidermoid carcinoma of the head and neck. Am J Surg 130:481–486
Taylor SG, Applebaum E, Showel JL et al. (1985) A randomized trial of adjuvant chemotherapy in head and neck cancer. J Clin Oncol 3:672–679
Toohill RJ, Anderson T, Byhardt RW et al. (1987) Cisplatin and fluorouracil as neoadjuvant therapy in head and neck cancer. Arch Otolaryngol Head Neck Surg 113:758–761
Urba SG, Forastiere AA, Wolf GT et al. (1989) Neoadjuvant chemotherapy with high dose continuous infusion cisplatin, 5-fluorouracil and mitoguazone for head and neck cancer. Proc Am Soc Clin Oncol 8:172
Urba SG, Wolf GT, McLaughlin P, Hazuka M (1992) Neoadjuvant carboplatin, 5-fluorouracil and radiation therapy for organ preservation in patients with resectable advanced head and neck cancer. 3rd international conference on head neck cancer, San Francisco, July 1992
Vokes EE, Schulsky RL, Weichselbaum RR et al. (1990) Induction chemotherapy with cisplatin, fluorouracil and high dose leucovorin for locally advanced head and neck cancer: a clinical and pharmacologic analysis. J Clin Oncol 8:241–247
Volling P, Schroder M, Rausching W et al. (1989) Carboplatin: the better platinum in head and neck cancer. Arch Otolaryngol Head Neck Surg 115:695–698
Weaver A, Flemming S, Kish J et al. (1982) Cisplatin and 5-fluorouracil as induction therapy for advanced head and neck cancer. Am J Surg 144:445–448
Wolf GT (1984) An overview of preoperative chemotherapy: where do we go from here? Am J Otolaryngol 5:77–79
Wolf GT, Fisher SG (1992) Effectiveness of salvage neck dissection for advanced regional metastases when induction chemotherapy and radiation are used for organ preservation. Laryngoscope 102:(in press)

Carcinomas of the Oropharynx Treated with Hyperfractionated Radiation Therapy on Radiation Therapy Oncology Group Protocol 8313

K.K. Fu[1], J.D. Cox[2], T.F. Pajak[3], V.A. Marcial[4], L.R. Coia[5], M. Mohiuddin[6], H.M. Selim[7], R.W. Byhardt[8], S. McDonald[9], H.G. Ortiz[10], and L. Martin[3]

[1] University of California, San Francisco, Radiation Oncology L-08, 505 Parnassus Avenue, San Francisco, CA 94143-0226, USA
[2] M.D. Anderson Cancer Center, 1515 Holcombe Boulevard, Houston, TX 77030, USA
[3] Radiation Therapy Oncology Group Headquarters, American College of Radiology, 1101 Market Street, 14th Floor, Philadelphia, PA 19107, USA
[4] Radiation Oncology Center, G.P.O. Box 70321, San Juan, PR 00936, USA
[5] Fox Chase Cancer Center, Philadelphia, PA 19111, USA
[6] Department of Rad Ther-Bodine Center, Thomas Jefferson University Hospital, Eleventh & Walnut Streets, Philadelphia, PA 19107, USA
[7] Department of Radiation Therapy, The Methodist Hospital, 506 6th Street, Brooklyn, NY 11215, USA
[8] Department of Radiologic Therapy, Zablocki V.A. Hospital, 5000 W. National Avenue, Milwaukee, WI 53295, USA
[9] Department of Radiation Oncology, University of Rochester, 601 Elmwood Avenue, Box 647, Rochester, NY 14643, USA
[10] Department of Radiological Sciences, Puerto Rico Cancer Center, G.P.O. Box 5067, San Juan, PR 00936, USA

Introduction

Squamous cell carcinomas of the oropharynx are among the sites within the upper aerodigestive tract most consistently treated with radiation therapy. The ability to observe directly the response to radiation therapy and to document local-regional control and failure result in their being excellent sites to investigate modifiers of radiation effects.

The last decade has seen a number of clinical trials pursuing altered fractionation. One of these trials, reported by Horiot et al. (1992) on behalf of the Radiotherapy Group of the European Organization for Research on Treatment of Cancer (EORTC), has suggested a benefit from hyperfractionated radiation therapy for small to moderately sized oropharyngeal squamous cell carcinomas, excluding carcinomas of the base of tongue. The Radiation Therapy Oncology Group (RTOG) completed a series of prospective, randomized Phase I_{LE}/II studies of hyperfractionated radiotherapy (Diener-West et al. 1991). One of these, RTOG Protocol 83-13, dealt with carcinomas of the upper respiratory and digestive tracts (Cox et al. 1990b, 1991; Cox et al. 1992). In this report, we have analyzed specifically the results in patients with carcinomas of the oropharynx and compared them to the results of the EORTC phase III trial (Horiot et al. 1992).

Materials and Methods

The rationale, eligibility criteria, evaluation parameters, radiation dose specifications, fractionation, end points, and statistical considerations have been published previously (Cox et al. 1990b). Patients were stratified by performance status, site of the primary tumor, and presence or absence of clinically positive cervical lymph node metastasis, and then allocated to one of three treatment arms of hyperfractionated radiotherapy: 67.2 Gy, 72.0 Gy, or 76.8 Gy. After sufficient evidence of tolerance at the 76.8 Gy level was available, the 81.6 Gy arm was opened and the 67.2 Gy arm was closed. Fractions of 1.2 Gy were given twice daily, 5 days per week. The interval between fractions each day was permitted to vary from 4 to 8 h (the actual treatment time was recorded).

Patients were considered to have complete tumor clearance when complete disappearance of the tumor at the primary site and any palpable lymph nodes had occurred. Estimates of local-regional control rates for patients who did not achieve an initial complete clearance were considered treatment failures on the first day of the study; patients who achieved initial complete clearance were considered treatment failures when a recurrence either at the primary or nodal sites was reported. For survival analysis, patients who died, regardless of the cause of death, were considered treatment failures.

Radiation-induced normal tissue effects were considered acute if the toxicity related to treatment occurred within the first 90 days from the start of treatment, and late if they persisted beyond 90 days or first occurred beyond day 90. The toxicities were scored from 0 (none) to 5 (fatal) (Cox et al. 1990).

A comprehensive reevaluation of the treatment actually delivered was completed by the study chair prior to analysis of results. Criteria for compliance with respect to the margins of the fields, total dose, fractionation, and total elapsed time were established. An overall time of 4 days beyond that allowed by the protocol was considered as "per protocol." Thus, 5 or more days beyond the treatment time specified for the particular total dose arm was considered a deviation (Cox et al. 1992).

Differences in the treatment delivery parameters (dose and time) between two patient groups were evaluated by the chi-squared test. Differences in the distributions of local-regional control and survival were evaluated by the Mantel-Haenszel (log rank) test (Mantel 1966). All the reported significance levels were based on a two-sided test. The time events were plotted as step functions using the Kaplan-Meier product-limit method

(Kaplan and Meier 1958). The various rates reported at 1, 2, and 3 years were based on the Kaplan-Meier estimates. Time was measured from the start of treatment until time of the first failure, or last follow-up if the patient did not fail.

Results

A total of 479 patients were randomized, of which 30 were cancelled, ineligible, or had no data available. Thus, 449 patients were evaluable for the end points of the trial. Of these, 193 patients had squamous cell carcinomas arising from oropharyngeal structures.

Table 1 shows the T and N stage distribution by the classification of the American Joint Committee on Cancer (1983) for the entire group of 193 patients. In order to achieve greater homogeneity and greater comparability with the experiences of the EORTC Radiotherapy Group phase III trial (Horiot et al. 1992), the 57 patients who had T2–3 N0–1 disease were identified as a subset and referred to as group 1. The rest of the patients were referred to as group 2 (T1–3 N2–3 and T4 N0–3) and the entire group as group 0. Thus group 1 represented the patients with more favorable stage II (two patients) and stage III (55 patients) lesions, and group 2 included patients with more extensive stage IV disease. The comparisons of pretreatment characteristics of these groups are shown in Table 2.

Table 3 characterizes these patients with regard to the treatment delivered. A significantly greater proportion of patients in group 1 received the dose per protocol than those in group 2 ($p = 0.02$). There were also significantly less treatment delays in group 1 ($p = 0.03$).

Local-regional control at 3 years is shown in Table 4. There was a trend towards higher local-regional control for the upper three doses compared to the lowest total dose (67.2 Gy) arm. Although the difference was not significant ($p = 0.12$), there was a significant difference in 3-year local-regional control between group 1 and group 2 (63% vs. 27%, $p = 0.0001$). Delay in

Table 1. Radiation Therapy Oncology Group Protocol 83-13: squamous cell carcinomas of the oropharynx (distribution by T and N stage)

T Stage	N stage			
	N0	N1	N2	N3
T1	0	0	2	4
T2	2	12	9	1
T3	26	17	25	35
T4	13	12	15	20

Table 2. Radiation Therapy Oncology Group Protocol 83-13: squamous cell carcinomas of the oropharynx (pretreatment characteristics)

	Group 0[a]	Group 1[b]	Group 2[c]
Number of patients	193	57	136
Male : Female	3.1 : 1	3.4 : 1	3 : 1
Age (years)			
Median	62	62	61
Range	22–85	44–85	22–85
KPS			
90–100	104 (54%)	35 (62%)	69 (51%)
70–80	73 (38%)	19 (33%)	54 (40%)
50–60	16 (8%)	3 (5%)	13 (9%)
Region			
Faucial arch	23 (12%)	8 (14%)	15 (11%)
Tonsillar fossa	61 (32%)	19 (33%)	42 (31%)
Base of tongue	62 (32%)	15 (26%)	47 (34%)
Pharyngeal wall	14 (7%)	5 (9%)	9 (7%)
Oropharynx, NOS	33 (17%)	10 (18%)	23 (17%)

KPS, Karnofsky performance scale; NOS, not otherwise specified.
[a] Group 0 (group 1 + group 2), T1–4 N0–3.
[b] Group 1, T2–3 N0–1 (stages II and III).
[c] Group 2, T1–3 N2–3 and T4 N0–3 (stage IV).

Table 3. Radiation Therapy Oncology Group Protocol 83-13: squamous cell carcinomas of the oropharynx (treatment delivery)

	Group 0[a]	Group 1[b]	Group 2[c]
Number of patients	193	57	136
Assigned total dose			
67.2 Gy	30 (15%)	10 (17%)	20 (15%)
72.0 Gy	60 (31%)	21 (37%)	39 (29%)
76.8 Gy	44 (23%)	8 (14%)	36 (26%)
81.6 Gy	59 (31%)	18 (32%)	41 (30%)
Dose delivered			
Per protocol	163 (85%)	54 (95%)	109 (80%)
Minor variations	7 (4%)	1 (2%)	6 (4%)
Major variations	22 (11%)	2 (3%)	21 (16%)
		($p = 0.02$)	
Treatment delays	$n = 163$	$n = 54$	$n = 109$
(Per protocol total dose only)			
+1–4 days	112 (69%)	43 (80%)	69 (63%)
+5–9 days	19 (12%)	2 (4%)	17 (16%)
+10–13 days	12 (7%)	3 (5%)	9 (8%)
≥14 days	20 (12%)	6 (11%)	14 (13%)
		($p = 0.03$)	

[a] Group 0 (group 1 + group 2), T1–4 N0–3.
[b] Group 1, T2–3 N0–1 (stages II and III).
[c] Group 2, T1–3 N2–3 and T4 N0–3 (stage IV).

Table 4. Radiation Therapy Oncology Group Protocol 83-13: squamous cell carcinomas of the oropharynx (3-year local-regional control)

	3-Year local-regional control Group 0[b]	Group 1[c]	Group 2[e]
No. of patients	193	57	136
All doses	38%	63%	27%
67.2 Gy	24%	–[d]	18%
Upper three doses	40%	69%	28%
	($p = 0.12$)	–[d]	($p = 0.38$)
Average daily interfraction interval			
<4.5 h	35%	56%	27%
≥4.5 h	40%	69%	28%
	($p = 0.36$)	($p = 0.38$)	($p = 0.60$)
Treatment delays[a]			
Per protocol	49%	71%	35%
≥5 days	27%	33%	25%
	($p = 0.004$)	($p = 0.05$)	($p = 0.11$)

[a] Patients required to survive 90+ days.
[b] Group 0 (group 1 + group 2), T1–4 N0–3.
[c] Group 1, T2–3 N0–1 (stages II and III).
[d] Only ten patients – too small a sample for reliable estimate or comparison.
[e] Group 2, T1–3 N2–3 and T4 N0–3 (stage IV).

completion of treatment was identified as an important prognostic factor for local-regional control among the patients who received their treatments "per protocol" with respect to total dose, target volume, and fractionation. The 3-year local-regional control was 49%, 71%, and 35% for patients treated per protocol and 27%, 33%, and 25% for those with delays of 5 or more days for groups 0, 1, and 2, respectively (p = 0.004, 0.05, and 0.11).

There was no significant difference in survival between the upper three total dose arms and the lowest dose arm (Fig. 1). However, treatment delays had a significant impact on survival. As shown in Fig. 2, survival for the entire group was significantly worse in patients with treatment delays of 5 or more days than for those who were treated per protocol ($p = 0.04$). The survival of patients in the more favorable group 1 was related only to delay in completion of treatment (3-year survival of 58% for delays of less than 5 days vs. 18% for delays of 5 or more days, $p = 0.06$). Similar to local-regional control, the 3-year survival was also significantly better in group 1 than in group 2 (51% vs. 27%, $p = 0.003$).

Severe (RTOG grade 4) late effects were infrequent. The cumulative probabilities of late effects at 1, 2, and 3 years were not significantly different among the four total dose arms (Table 5). Average daily interfraction interval had a significant impact on the development of late effects. An estimated 10% of patients had severe late effects at 3 years when the average daily interfraction interval was less than 4.5 h, compared with only

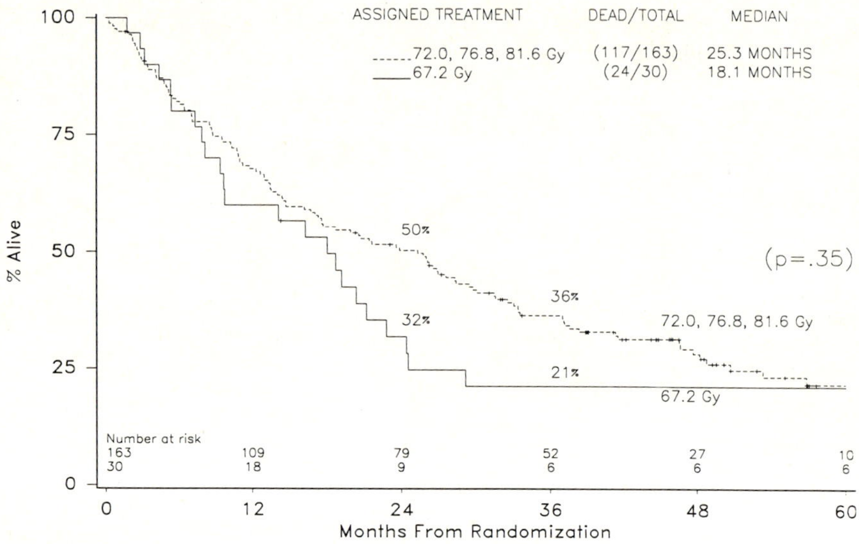

Fig. 1. Radiation Therapy Oncology Group Protocol 8313: overall survival curves for all patients as a function of dose (oropharynx patients only)

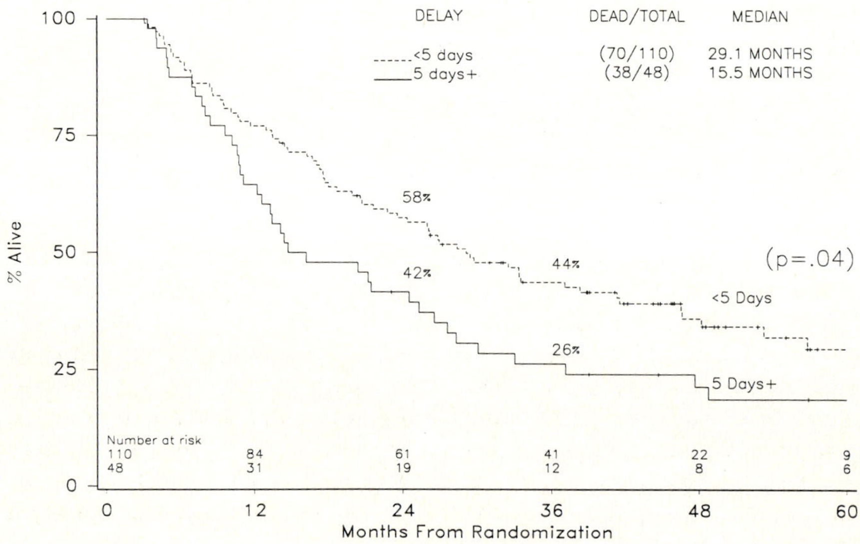

Fig. 2. Radiation Therapy Oncology Group Protocol 8313: overall survival curves for all patients as a function of treatment delay (oropharynx patients only)

Table 5. Radiation Therapy Oncology Group Protocol 83-13: squamous cell carcinomas of the oropharynx (severe late effects)[a]

Patient group	Late effects/patients	Cumulative probability 1 Year	2 Years	3 Years
All doses	8/173[c]	4%	4%	5%
67.2 Gy	0/28	0%	0%	0%
72.0 Gy	3/54	4%	4%	8%
76.8 Gy	2/38	6%	6%	6%
81.6 Gy	3/53[c]	4%	4%	4%
Average daily interfraction interval				
<4.5 h	7/82[c]	7%	7%	10%
≥4.5 h	1/91	1%	1%	1%
			(p = 0.02)	
Treatment delays[b]				
Per protocol	6/110[c]	4%	4%	6%
≥5 days	2/48	5%	5%	5%

[a] Necroses of soft tissue or bone. (20 patients who died before 90 days were excluded from analysis.)
[b] Patients required to survive 90+ days.
[c] One toxicity occurred at 46.8 months.

1% when it was 4.5 h or longer ($p = 0.02$). Delay in completion of protocol had no influence on the probability of late effects.

Discussion

The primary rationale for hyperfractionated radiotherapy is that with decrease of dose per fraction, it is possible to increase the total dose, thereby increasing tumor control without increasing late normal tissue toxicity. In this phase I_{LE}/II dose escalation study of hyperfractionated radiotherapy, although there was a trend towards better local-regional control with increase of total dose from 67.2 Gy to doses of 72.0 Gy or more in the patients with squamous cell carcinoma of oropharynx, the difference was not statistically significant. It should be noted that this dose-escalating trial was not specifically designed to detect an increase in local-regional control for a particular region. In addition, the number of patients in each arm was too small to detect a difference. If all the sites are used in the analysis, the 67.2 Gy arm had significantly inferior local-regional control than the combined upper three doses ($p = 0.03$). We saw no increase of local-regional control with increase of dose to above 72.0 Gy. A similar "plateauing" phenomenon of dose–response relationship for total doses of 70–72 Gy or more was also observed in other RTOG phase I_{LE}/II dose escalation trials of hyperfractionated radiotherapy in non-small cell carcinoma of the lung (Cox et al.

1990a) and malignant gliomas (Nelson et al. 1993). The pretreatment patient characteristics with respect to Karnofsky performance status (KPS) and T and N stages appear well balanced for the different total dose arms. Treatment delivery in terms of dose delivered per protocol and elapsed days was also not significantly different for the different total dose arms. At the present time, the reason for the "plateauing" phenomenon for doses above 70–72 Gy with hyperfractionated radiation therapy remains uncertain.

The adverse effect of prolonged overall treatment time on treatment outcome in head and neck cancer patients have been demonstrated in a number of studies reported previously (Pajak et al. 1991; Cox et al. 1992); Parson et al. 1980; Overgaard et al. 1988; Keane et al. 1992). Presumably, this is due to tumor repopulation during treatment interruptions. Treatment delays may be particularly deleterious for tumors with short potential doubling times (T_{pot}) and when the interruptions occur late in the treatment course, when accelerated repopulation may take place (Withers et al. 1988). In general, the T_{pot} for head and neck cancers and in particular tonsillar carcinomas is relatively short (Fowler et al. 1990; Wilson et al. 1988). In this study, treatment delays of 5 or more days had an adverse effect on the local-regional control and survival, even in patients with more favorable stages of disease.

Stage of disease is clearly an important prognostic factor in local-regional control and survival in carcinoma of the oropharynx, as evidenced by the significantly better treatment outcome in group 1 patients with T2–3 N0–1 carcinomas of the oropharynx. In addition to a lesser tumor burden, patient compliance to protocol treatment was also significantly better in group 1 than in group 2. Better treatment tolerance and compliance might have contributed to the improved treatment outcome in these patients.

This study demonstrated that using hyperfractionated radiotherapy, total doses up to 81.6 Gy can be delivered with acceptable late normal tissue toxicity. The average interfraction interval between the two daily fractions had a significant impact on the probability of severe late toxicity, although it had no effect on the local-regional control or survival. This may be due to incomplete repair of sublethal damage for interfraction intervals shorter than 4.5 h (Rojas and Joiner 1989). We saw no dose–response relationship in the development of severe late toxicity among the four different total dose arms in this study. However, it should be noted that there was a greater proportion of patients with an average daily interfraction interval of 4.5 h or longer in the 81.6 Gy arm than in the other lower total dose arms (Cox et al. 1991). This might have been a factor in the low incidence of severe late toxicity in the 81.6 Gy arm. A daily interfraction interval of 6 h or longer has been adapted for all current RTOG trials using twice-daily fractionation schedules.

In this RTOG study, the local-regional control rate of hyperfractionated radiotherapy for patients with T2–3 N0–1 carcinomas of the oropharynx (group 1) are comparable to the results of the hyperfractionation arm of the

EORTC trial (Horiot et al. 1992). In contrast to the EORTC trial, this study was a phase I_{LE}/II trial and included patients with base of tongue primaries, which accounted for 32% of the patient population. The dose per fraction was slightly higher than that used in the EORTC trial, and a range of total doses from 67.2 Gy to 81.6 Gy were used. Assuming that $\alpha/\beta = 10$ Gy, the biologically effective dose (BED; Fowler 1992) would be 84 Gy_{10} for the conventional fractionation arm and 90 Gy_{10} for the hyperfractionation arm of the EORTC trial. The BED for the 67.2 Gy, 72.0 Gy, 76.8 Gy, and 81.6 Gy hyperfractionation arms of the RTOG trial would be 75 Gy_{10}, 81 Gy_{10}, 86 Gy_{10}, and 91 Gy_{10}, respectively. In this subset of patients (group 1), we also saw no dose–response relationship for local-regional control. The 3-year local-regional control rate was 63% for all dose arms and 69% for the upper three dose arms. In the EORTC trial, patients treated with hyperfractionated radiotherapy had significantly better local-regional control than those treated with conventional fractionated radiotherapy (Horiot et al. 1992). Whether hyperfractionated radiotherapy is better than conventional fractionated radiotherapy for patients with advanced carcinomas of various head and neck primary sites, including the oropharynx, and its relative efficacy in comparison to split-course accelerated hyperfractionated radiotherapy (Wang 1988) and accelerated fractionated radiotherapy, using a concomitant boost technique (Ang and Peters 1992), are currently under investigation in a four-arm randomized trial (Cox 1992).

References

Ang KK, Peters LJ (1992) Concomitant boost radiotherapy in the treatment of head and neck cancers. Semin Radiat Oncol 2:31–33

Cox JD (1992) Clinical perspectives of recent developments in fractionation. Semin Radiat Oncol 2:10–15

Cox JD, Azarnia N et al. (1990a) A randomized phase I/II trial of hyperfractionated radiation therapy with total doses of 60.0 Gy to 79.2 Gy: possible survival benefits with ≥69.6 Gy in favorable patients with Radiation Therapy Oncology Group stage III non-small-cell lung carcinoma: report of Radiation Therapy Oncology Group 82-11. J Clin Oncol 8:1543–1555

Cox JD, Pajak TF et al. (1990b) Dose–response for local control with hyperfractionated radiation therapy in advanced carcinomas of the upper aerodigestive tracts: preliminary report of Radiation Therapy Oncology Group Protocol 83-13. Int J Radiat Oncol Biol Phys 18:515–521

Cox JD, Pajak TF et al. (1991) ASTRO plenary: interfraction interval is a major determinant of late effects, with hyperfractionated radiation therapy of carcinomas of upper respiratory and digestive tracts: results from Radiation Therapy Oncology Group Protocol 8313. Int J Radiat Oncol Biol Phys 20:1191–1195

Cox JD, Pajak TF et al. (1992) Interruptions adversely affect local control and survival with hyperfractionated radiation therapy of carcinomas of the respiratory/digestive tracts: new evidence for accelerated proliferation from RTOG Protocol 8313. Cancer 69:2744–2748

Diener-West M, Pajak TF et al. (1991) Randomized dose-searching Phase I_{LE}/II trials of fractionation in radiation therapy for cancer. J Natl Cancer Inst 83: 1065–1071

Fowler JF, Tanner MA et al. (1990) Further analysis of the time factor in squamous cell carcinoma of the tonsillar region. Radiother Oncol 19:237–244

Fowler JF (1992) Brief summary of radiobiological principles in fractionated radiotherapy. Semin Radiat Oncol 2:16–21

Horiot JC, LeFur R et al. (1992) Status of the experience of the EORTC Cooperative Group of radiotherapy with hyperfractionated and accelerated radiotherapy regimes. Semin Radiat Oncol 2:34–37

Kaplan EL, Meier P (1958) Nonparametric estimation from incomplete observations. J Amer Stat Assoc 53:457–481

Keane TJ, Fyles A et al. (1992) The effect of treatment duration on local control of squamous cell carcinoma of the tonsil and carcinoma of the cervix. Semin Radiat Oncol 2:26–28

Mantel N (1966) Evaluation of survival data and two new rank order statistics arising in its consideration. Cancer Chem Rep 5:163–170

Nelson DF, Scott C et al. (1993) Hyperfractionated radiation therapy and BCNU in the treatment of malignant glioma; possible advantage observed at 72 Gy bid fractions: report of RTOG 8302. Int J Radiat Oncol Biol Phys 25:193–207

Overgaard J, Hjelm-Hansen M et al. (1988) Comparison of conventional and split-course radiotherapy as primary treatment in carcinoma of the larynx. Acta Oncol 27:147–152

Pajak TF, Laramore GE et al. (1991) Elapsed treatment days – a critical item for radiotherapy quality control review in head and neck trials: RTOG report. Int J Radiat Oncol Biol Phys 20:13–20

Parsons JT, Bova FJ et al. (1980) A re-evaluation of split-course technique for squamous cell carcinoma of the head and neck. Int J Radiat Oncol Biol Phys 6:1645–1652

Rojas A, Joiner MC (1989) The influence of dose per fraction on repair kinetics. Radiother Oncol 14:329–336

Wang CC (1988) Twice-daily radiation therapy for head and neck carcinomas. Front Radiat Ther Oncol 22:93–98

Wilson GD, McNally NJ et al. (1988) Measurement of cell kinetics in human tumors in vivo using BUdR in flow cytometry. Br J Cancer 58:423–431

Withers HR, Taylor JMG et al. (1988) The hazards of accelerated tumor clonogen repopulation during radiotherapy. Acta Oncol 27:131–146

Preoperative Radiochemotherapy and Radical Surgery of Advanced Head and Neck Cancers – Results of a Prospective, Multicenter DÖSAK Study

C. Mohr[1], W. Bohndorf[2], H. Gremmel[3], F. Härle [4], J.-E. Hausamen[5], H. Hirche[6], M. Molls[7], K.H. Renner[8], J. Reuther[9], H. Sack[7], D. Schettler[1], H. Scheunemann[10], and M. Thelen[11]

[1] Klinik für Gesichts- und Kieferchirurgie, Universitätsklinik Essen, Hufelandstr. 55, 45122 Essen, Germany
[2] Strahlenklinik, Universitätsklinik Würzburg, Pleicher Wall 2, 97070 Würzburg, Germany
[3] Strahlenklinik am Klinikum, Christian-Albrechts-Universität, Kiel, Arnold-Heller-Str. 5, 24105 Kiel, Germany
[4] Abteilung für Kieferchirurgie, Christian-Albrechts-Universität, Kiel, Arnold-Heller-Str. 5, 24105 Kiel, Germany
[5] Klinik und Poliklinik für Mund-Kiefer-Gesichtschirurgie, Medizinischen Hochschule, Konstanty-Gutschow-Str. 8, 30625 Hanover, Germany
[6] Institut für Medizinische Informatik und Biomathematik, Universitätsklinik Essen, Hufelandstr. 55, 45122 Essen, Germany
[7] Radiologisches Zentrum, Universität Essen, Hufelandstr. 55, 45122 Essen, Germany
[8] Strahlenklinik, Medizinischen Hochschule Hanover, Konstanty-Gutschow-Str. 8, 30625 Hanover, Germany
[9] Klinik und Poliklinik für Mund-Kiefer-Gesichtschirurgie, Universität Würzburg, Pleicher Wall 2, 97070 Würzburg, Germany
[10] Klinik für Mund-Kiefer-Gesichtschirurgie, Johannes Gutenberg-Universität Mainz, Langenbechstr. 1, 55131 Mainz, Germany
[11] Strahlenklinik, Johannes Gutenberg Universität Mainz, Langenbechstr. 1, 55131 Mainz, Germany

Introduction

Present research concerning the efficiacy of therapeutic strategies for squamous cell carcinomas of the oral cavity and the oropharynx profits from former observational studies. The so-called retrospective German, Austrian, and Swiss Association for Head and Neck Tumors (DÖSAK) study (Platz et al. 1986) served to review existing proposals for classification (UICC 1973, 1978; AJC 1978) and to develop a statistical classification which enables the head and neck oncologist to define prognostically homogeneous patient collectives. The treatment-dependent prognostic index (TPI) was the corresponding result (Platz et al. 1982).

The subsequent prospective DÖSAK study gave the opportunity of applying and analyzing this new classification on an independent patient collective. Despite minor differences from the first study, this prospective study confirmed the high degree of accuracy of the TPI to determine individual and collective prognoses (Platz et al. 1989). In consequence of these studies, the DÖSAK has proposed the TPI as an alternative to the Tumor Node Metastases (TNM) system, which does justice to the demands of clinical studies. The survival analysis of our following study therefore relates to this TPI classification.

The preceding two DÖSAK studies had failed to establish a positive effect of any combined treatment modality when compared with radical surgery alone. The appertaining survival curves after isolated surgical treatment are, therefore, suitable as a basis of evaluation for alternative treatment strategies. On the other hand, we had observed encouraging results with an interdisciplinary treatment regimen for incurable head and neck tumours in Essen (Schmitt et al. 1983). Therefore, our regional cooperative group decided to transfer this strategy to advanced, but operable, squamous cell carcinomas of the oral cavity and the oropharynx. The following results were obtained by prospective, multicenter, interdisciplinary cooperation of radiotherapists and maxillofacial surgeons at the Universities of Kiel, Hanover, Mainz, Würzburg, and Essen.

Material and Methods

From January 1985 to December 1987, 165 patients were entered into the study. The follow-up period lasted from March 1985 to May 1991. Only patients with advanced, primary, biopsy-proven squamous cell carcinomas of the oral cavity and the oropharynx without distant metastasis were eligible for the study. A minimal tumor size of 2 cm was required. The stage of regional lymph nodes was not fixed. Because of their supposed better prognosis, lip carcinomas were excluded. Only those patients in a condition to undergo radical surgical treatment and without contraindications against cisplatin were included in the study.

The preoperative treatment consisted of 32 Gy (5 × 2 Gy per week) from a supervoltage source, applied to the primary tumor and to both sides of the neck as far as the clavicles. During the first week of treatment, the patients also received cisplatin in a daily dose of 20 mg/m^2 body surface. Radical surgery was carried out after a delay of 10–14 days.

Complete, prospectively documented data were centrally collected in Essen and analyzed in the following manner: first, a descriptive evaluation of all data consisting of one-dimensional frequency counts and cross tables was performed. Second, the prognostic relevance of each clinical, therapeutic, and histopathological factor according to recurrence and survival was investigated in isolation. For graphic presentation, the product-limit method was selected (Kaplan and Meier 1958). Comparison of survival curves was performed by the Gehan-Wilcoxon test and the log rank test (Gehan 1965; Mantel 1966; Cox 1972).

After obtaining prior information by this univariate analysis, a multivariate assessment of all potentially important factors was carried out by means of the regression analysis model of Cox (1972). Thus, the real prognostic influence and significance of each clinical, pathological, or therapeutic factor became clear. The significance level was set at 95% in all analyses.

For comparison of the survival rates obtained by our combined treatment modalities, each patient was associated with his or her individual TPI. This enabled us to compare the observed outcome of our patients after combined treatment modalities with the corresponding "estimated survival rates" (Platz et al. 1986) for the same patients treated with surgery alone and with the factual survival of those patients in the retrospective DÖSAK study, for whom the prognostic factors were the same. Finally, we did the same with the corresponding data of the prospective DÖSAK study (Platz et al. 1989).

Results

The ratio of male to female patients was 5:1. The patients ranged in age from 30 to 78 years, with an average age of 53 years (Table 1). Fixed date for evaluation was the April 30, 1991. A total of 37 patients had suffered from local or regional recurrence, 22 distant metastases or secondary malignomas in distant sites had developed, and 66 patients (40%) had died during the follow-up period. Despite the fact that 31 patients had died

Table 1. Characteristics and results of prospective, multicenter study

Number of patients	165
Treatment period	01/1985–12/1987
Follow-up period	03/1985–05/1991
Average age	53 years
Male (*n*)	137
Female (*n*)	28
Therapeutic effect	
a) No evidence of disease	157 (95%)
b) Evidence of disease	8 (5%)
Recurrent disease	
a) Locoregional	37 (22%)
b) Distant metastasis	22 (13%)
Died during follow-up period	
a) Of carcinoma	31 (19%)
b) Intercurrent disease	35 (21%)
Alive through follow-up period	99 (60%)
Lost during follow-up period	3 (2%)

unrelated to their squamous cell carcinoma, we considered the cause of death in all 66 patients to be the tumor in the life table calculations. We selected this procedure to allow comparison of the survival rates with the retrospective and prospective DÖSAK studies. Only three patients were lost to follow-up.

In *univariate analysis*, each factor was considered by itself and isolated from the others. We could not establish a significant relevance of the patients' sex, age, or tumor site. This was true irrespective of differentiation between oral cavity and oropharynx, locostable and mobile tumor sites, or precanine, postcanine, and postmolar locations. However, lip carcinomas were excluded from the study by the protocol. Interestingly, univariate analysis revealed a significant influence for the delay between the beginning of the irradiation and the operation. An overall treatment time exceeding 50 days deteriorated the prognosis. The degree of histological differentiation also proved relevant. Poorly differentiated tumors led to an impaired chance of survival. On the whole, the TPI was significantly related to the clinical outcome of the patients.

As in former evaluations, the histopathological findings after the preoperative treatment turned out to be the most important prognostic factors. If the pathologist could not establish evidence of living tumor cells within the removed primary or within the dissected regional lymph nodes after the preoperative irradiation, the prognosis was significantly better (Mohr et al. 1990).

The simultaneous, competitive assessment of all investigated factors by means of *multivariate analysis* reduced the number of factors relevant to the prognosis to three (Table 2):

1. The histopathological demonstration of active tumor cells within the removed neck nodes exceeded the influence of the clinical degree of lymph node fixation and showed a significant influence below a p value of 1%. This result was not surprising because only 42% of the clinically fixed lymph nodes showed evidence of tumor infiltration.
2. Complete devitalization of the primary led to a significant improvement of the chances of survival.
3. The Cox model confirmed the univariate finding of a significant influence of the histopathological grading, when comparing poorly differentiated carcinomas, which were in the minority, with highly or intermediately differentiated tumors, which were in the majority in our study. It became obvious by this multivariate analysis that the remaining clinical factors, which were significant in univariate analysis, were of minor importance for the prognosis.

As mentioned above, the documentation included all clinical factors required for the determination of the individual TPI of each patient. Depending on the kind of treatment and the therapeutic effect, the TPI provides an estimation for the survival of the respective single patient or the re-

Table 2. Results of multivariate analysis of all chinical, therapeutic, and histopathological data

Maximal tumor size	I a) <40 mm b) >40 mm	II Continual	Not significant
Regional lymph nodes	I a) Not palpable b) Palpable, moveable c) Palpable, fixed	II a) Palpable, fixed b) Not palpable or palpable moveable	Not significant
Site by organs	I a) Precanine b) Postcanine c) Postmolar	II a) Oropharynx b) Tongue c) Oral cavity	Not significant
Grading	I a) Grading I+II b) Grading III		$p < 0.01$
Sex	a) Male b) Female		Not significant
Age	I a) <50 years b) 50–70 years c) >70 years	II Continual	Not significant
Therapeutic effect	a) Evidence of disease b) No evidence of disease		Not significant
Histology of the removed tumor	a) Evidence of living tumor cells b) No evidence of living tumor cells		$p < 0.05$
Histology of the removed lymph nodes	a) Evidence of living tumor cells b) No evidence of living tumor cells		$p < 0.01$
Delay between beginning of irradiation and surgery	Continual		Not significant

According to the survival rate, histopathology of the primary tumor and the regional lymph nodes as well as the histopathological grading were the most important prognostic factors.

I, II, Variables used with the multivariate analysis. This was important because the different classification systems used, e.g. for tumor site, could have significantly influenced prognosis.

a,b,c, Variables analyzed using the Cox model.

spective collective. Therefore, we were able to directly compare our observations after combined treatment with the TPI estimations for the same patients after surgery alone. According to the amount and the compound of each TPI group, more or less considerable differences could be established between the observed survival and the TPI estimations.

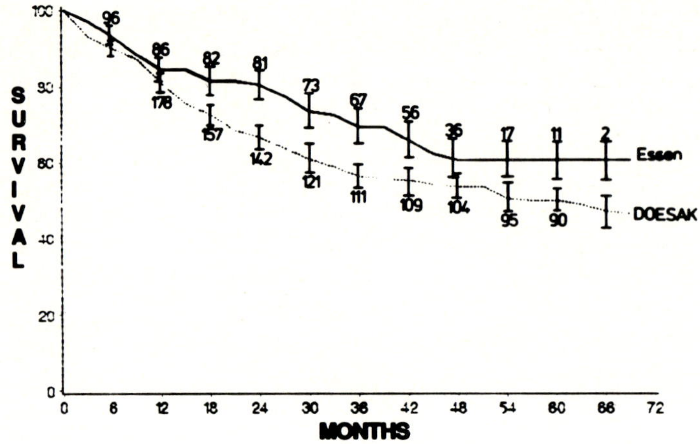

Fig. 1. Comparison of the survival curves after multimodality treatment (our study, "Essen"; *continuous line*; $n = 104$) and after radical surgery alone (retrospective DÖSAK study, "DÖSAK"; *dotted line*; $n = 234$). The significant prognostic amelioration is attributed to the preoperative treatment ($p < 0.05$)

In order to obtain a reliable assessment concerning the prognostic benefit of our preoperative treatment strategy, we compared our survival observations with the corresponding patients in the retrospective DÖSAK study. Four TPI groups were represented as well in the DÖSAK study as in our study. These four groups (TPI values E 38-A-NED, E 15-A-NED, E 14-A-NED, and E 13-A-NED) consisted of deeply infiltrating tumors of 0–4 cm (E 15-A-NED, E 14-A-NED, and E 13-A-NED) or more than 4 cm (E 38-A-NED) in various age-groups. (*A* refers to treatment group A who underwent radical surgery, and *NED* means no evidence of disease.)

104 patients after combined treatment in our study were compared with 234 patients after radical surgery alone in the retrospective DÖSAK study. After a follow-up period of 6 years, we established a statistically significant difference between the two treatment strategies. The patients in our study showed a significantly better prognosis, which we attributed to the preoperative irradiation and adjuvant cisplatin therapy (Fig. 1).

The differences between the survival rates clearly emerged during the second postoperative year, reaching maximum values of nearly 14% during the second, third, and fourth year and amounting to 10% 5 years after treatment. The differences were statistically significant in the Gehan-Wilcoxon test as well as the log rank test.

Discussion

With regard to the expected small prognostic ameliorations, comparison between two different strategies for the treatment of squamous cell carcinomas of the oral cavity and oropharynx requires a large series of patients (Peto et al. 1976). On the other hand, the well-known low incidence of this tumor impedes accumulation of great numbers of patients, even in multicenter studies.

Because of the small patient collectives, the majority of randomized trials fail to provide statistically supported results (Freyman et al. 1978). Therefore, reports about considerable prognostic ameliorations by surgical (Hemprich 1987) or multimodality treatment strategies (Holm et al. 1983; Müller et al. 1985; Knöbber et al. 1987) have to be interpreted with prudence. Different procedures for the assessment of dead patients further complicate any attempt at comparison. Additionally, existing, exclusively clinical classifications such as TNM (UICC 1978) or tumor stage (AJC 1978) are not suitable to guarantee a prognostically homogeneous distribution of the patients.

In 1982, SIMON stated that the prior condition for performing clinical trials is a statistical prognostic classification for the tumor of interest. The TPI presented by DÖSAK (Platz et al. 1982, 1986) has proved to be a feasible method of meeting this demand.

Based on the TPI classification, we observed a considerable difference between the survival curves after our combined treatment and after surgery alone. Despite this statistically proven difference, the results have to be interpreted with certain reservations regarding the comparison of our prospective data material with the historical data of the retrospective and prospective DÖSAK studies. Therefore a critical verification of the results by an independently acquired patient collective is of major importance.

The prospective DÖSAK study (Platz et al. 1989) provided this required collective in an ideal manner. Naturally, we were primarily interested in the four respective TPI groups which were represented in our study as well as the retrospective DÖSAK study, which the TPI is based on. Because of their relatively common constellation of prognostic clinical factors, the authors of the TPI reported a comparison for these four groups between the TPI estimations and the real survival rates within the prospective DÖSAK study (Platz et al. 1989).

Regarding the TPI groups E 38-A-NED and E 15-A-NED, they observed considerable differences between the survival rates within the prospective DÖSAK study. In our study, lip carcinomas were excluded. Therefore, the TPI estimations tended to be too favorable relative to our patients. Additionally, the TPI groups E 13-A-NED and E 14-A-NED in our study consisted of more extended tumours in prognostically less favorable sites compared with the retrospective DÖSAK study.

The results of the prospective DÖSAK study thus confirm our statistical findings of an ameliorated prognosis for patients after the combined treatment regimen. Nevertheless, critical evaluation of these results is required. Since 1989, we have, therefore, undertaken a multicenter, interdisciplinary, prospective, randomized trial to verify the benefit of our preoperative treatment strategy. Radical surgery according to the DÖSAK definitions (1982) alone will be compared with preoperative radiochemotherapy with only slight modifications also followed by radical surgery. The preliminary results confirm the assumption of a real benefit from the multimodality treatment.

Conclusion

From 1985 to 1987, 165 patients with advanced primary squamous cell carcinomas of the oral cavity and the oropharynx were treated by a multimodality strategy. In accordance with the recommendations of DÖSAK, each patient was classified according to his or her TPI (Platz et al. 1986). Preoperatively, the primary tumor and both sides of the neck were irradiated with a dose of 32 Gy (5 × 2 Gy per week). During the first week of treatment, the patients also received cisplatin in a daily dose of 20 mg/m^2 body surface. After a delay of 10–14 days, radical surgery was carried out. By means of multivariate analysis, a significant influence on the prognosis was demonstrated for the tumor and lymph node histopathology after the preoperative treatment.

Based on the TPI classification, the observed outcome of the patients after the combined treatment concept was compared with the survival of the corresponding patients of the retrospective DÖSAK study (Platz et al. 1986), which had been treated by surgery alone. A statistically proven amelioration of the survival was observed. The differences between the survival rates clearly emerged during the second postoperative year, reaching maximum values of nearly 14% during the second, third, and fourth year and amounting to 10% 5 years after treatment.

References

American Joint Committee for Cancer Staging and End Results Reporting (AJC) (1978) Manual for staging of cancer 1978. Chicago

Cox DR (1972) Regression models and life tables (with discussion). J R Stat Soc 34:187–220

DÖSAK (1982) Definitionen zum radikalchirurgischen Vorgehen bei Plattenepithelkarzinomen der Mundhöhle. Dtsch Z Mund-Kiefer-Gesichtschirc 6:369–372

Freyman JA, Chalmers TC, Smith H (1978) The importance of beta, the type II error and sample size in the design and interpretation of the randomized controlled trial. N Engl J Med 290:690

Gehan EA (1965) A generalized Wilcoxon test for comparing arbitrarily simply-censored samples. Biometrika 52:203–224

Hemprich A (1987) 15 Jahre radikale Neckdissection an der Kieferklinik der Universität Münster. Dtsch Z Mund Kiefer Gesichtschir 11:341–346

Holm LE, Lundquist PG, Silfverswärd C, Ruden BI, Sobin A, Wersäll J (1983) Combined preoperative radiotherapy and surgery in the treatment of carcinoma of the anterior two thirds of the tongue. Laryngoscope 93:792–796

Kaplan EL, Meier P (1958) Nonparametric estimation from incomplete observation J Am Stat Ass 53:457–481

Knöbber D, Sack H, Stützer H, Rose K (1987) Vorbestrahlung und Operation von Patienten mit einem Plattenepithelkarzinom der Mundhöhle und des Oropharynx: Ergebnisse einer Studie 1973–1984. Strahlenther Onkol 163:706–713

Mantel N (1966) Evaluation of survival data and two new rank order statistics arising in its consideration. Cancer Chemother Rep 50:163–170

Mohr CH, Bohndorf W, Gremmel H, Härle F, Hausamen JE, Hirche H, Molls M, Renner KH, Reuther J, Sack H, Schettler D, Scheunemann H, Thelen M (1990) Präoperative Radiation, cis Platin Sensibilisierung und radikale Resektion primär operabler Mundhöhlenkarzinome – Ergebnisse einer prospektiven Therapiestudie des DÖSAK. Dtsch Z Mund-Kiefer-Gesichtschir 14:242–249

Müller RP, Schärtel L, Hemprich A, Moring R (1985) Behandlungsergebnisse nach Strahlentherapie primär maligner Unterkiefertumoren. Dtsch Z Mund Kiefer Gesichtschir 9:83–88

Peto R, Pike M, Armitage P, Breslow N, Cox D, Howard S, Mantel N, Mc Pherson K, Peto J, Smith P (1976) Design and analysis of randomized clinical trials requiring prolonged observation of each patient: 1. Introduction and design. Br J Cancer 34:585

Platz H, Fries R, Hudec M (1982) Therapieabhängiger Prognoseindex TPI für Karzinome der Lippen, der Mundhöhle und des Oropharynx. Eigenvervielfältigung, Linz

Platz H, Fries R, Hudec M (1986) Prognoses of oral cavity carcinomas. Results of a multicentric retrospective observation study. Hanser, Munich

Platz H, Fries R, Hudec M (1989) Kritische Validierung des therapieabhängigen Prognoseindex TPI anhand der prospektiven DÖSAK-Studie über Plattenepithelkarzinome der Lippen, der Mundhöhle und des Oropharynx. Dtsch Z Mund-Kiefer-Gesichtschir 13:329–337

Schmitt G, Schettler D, Scheerer E, Higi M, Hauenstein HG (1983) Present interdisciplinary treatment regimen for advanced head and neck tumours at the West German Tumour Centre, Essen. J Max Fac Surg 11:51–53

Simon R (1982) Randomized clinical trials and research strategy. Cancer Treat Rep 66:1083–1087

UICC (1973) TNM Classification of malignant tumours. UICC, Geneva

UICC (1978) TNM Atlas. UICC, Geneva

Simultaneous Preoperative Radiochemotherapy with Cisplatin in Advanced Oral Cavity Carcinomas: Acute Response and Follow-Up

R.-P. Müller[1], S. Staar[1], M. Samek[2], and H.-D. Pape[2]

[1] Klinik und Poliklinik für Strahlentherapie, Mund-, Kiefer- und Gesichtschirurgie, Universität zu Köln, Joseph-Stelzmann-Str. 9, 50931 Cologne, Germany
[2] Zahn-, Mund- und Kieferheilkunde, Mund-, Kiefer- und Gesichtschirurgie, Universität zu Köln, Joseph-Stelzmann-Str. 9, 50931 Cologne, Germany

In order to test efficiency and feasibility, 136 patients with histologically proven squamous cell carcinomas of the oral cavity (T2–4 N0–3 M_0) were entered from January 1986 to October 1991 into a trial of preoperative simultaneous radiochemotherapy with cisplatin followed by radical surgery. End points of the study were local recurrence and survival.

Radiotherapy to the primary and regional lymph nodes was performed with fractions of 1.8 Gy daily up to a total dose of 39.6 Gy over 4.5 weeks. Chemotherapy consisted of 20 mg cisplatin/m^2 body surface area given intravenously on days 1–5 in week 1. Two weeks after the end of radiochemotherapy, patients with complete (CR) or partial remission (PR) underwent radical surgery and those with no change or progressive disease continued radiotherapy up to 70.2 Gy to the primary and 56–60 Gy to the lymph nodes, combined with a second course of cisplatin.

All patients were evaluable. Before therapy, 21% had stage II, 46% stage III, and 33% stage IV disease. Median age was 57 years, and the ratio of women to men was 1:4. After 39.6 Gy and 100 mg cisplatin/m^2, 45 out of 136 patients showed clinical CR and 37 patients had no tumor in the surgical specimen. A total of 94% could be downstaged. The actuarial 2-year survival rate is 84%, the 3-year survival rate 79%. The local recurrence rate after 2 years is 15%. This protocol reveals high effectiveness of preoperative simultaneous radiochemotherapy with cisplatin in advanced oral cavity carcinomas.

Introduction

Advanced oral cavity and oropharynx carcinomas continue to be a problem of local control. As many as one half or more of patients show local or regional recurrences, mainly during the first 2 years after initial treatment, and local failure often causes death (Fletcher 1983; Glanzmann 1978; Kutzner et al. 1982; Mendenhall et al. 1987; Vikram et al. 1980). Traditionally, these carcinomas have been treated with surgery and/or radiotherapy. Although radiation of this region is tolerable even in high doses, and in spite of improved radiation techniques, the large T3 and T4 cancers are more difficult to eradicate by local measures. Regional lymph node metastases are both a function of primary tumor site and size. For patients with oral cavity and oropharyngeal carcinomas T2 and greater, the incidence of microscopic or clinically evident lymph node metastasis is more than 50% (Fletcher 1980; Mendenhall et al. 1987). The search for new treatment schemes has been intensified during recent years. One way was the combination of chemotherapy, radiotherapy, and surgery. Most encouraging data were reported with a combined treatment using cisplatin alone or regimens containing cisplatin and simultaneous radiation (Dewitt 1987; Douple 1979; Jacobs 1984; Zamboglou et al. 1988). Cisplatin in combination with simultaneous radiation was used to achieve a radiation-sensitizing effect and to potentiate cell damage. Based on promising results obtained by Gefeller et al. (1985) and Schmitt et al. (1983) with radiochemotherapy using cisplatin in oral cavity carcinomas, in 1986 the Departments of Radiation Oncology and Maxilla-Facial Surgery at the University of Cologne initiated a protocol of preoperative simultaneous radiochemotherapy with cisplatin followed by radical surgery for advanced squamous cell carcinomas of the oral cavity.

Materials and Methods

Since 1986, 136 patients have been treated according to the protocol. All patients had histologically proven squamous cell carcinomas of the oral cavity in advanced stage without prior radio- or chemotherapy or surgery. Based on Union Internationale Contre le Cancer (UICC) classification (1987), 80% of the patients had stage III and IV disease. None had clinically evident distant metastases (Fig. 1). Most tumors were located in the floor of mouth, the lower alveolus, and the tongue (Fig. 2). Patients' characteristics revealed heavy smokers in 85% and alcoholics in 60%. Median age was 57 years, and the ratio of women to men was 1:4.

After complete staging including biopsy with tatooing of the tumor margins, ultrasound or computed tomography (CT)/magnetic resonance imaging (MRI) of the neck, laboratory examinations with complete blood count and biochemical survey, and exclusion of distant metastases by chest X-ray, liver ultrasound, and bone scan, patients were entered to the combined therapy protocol. Before radiochemotherapy was begun, all patients had an intensive dental evaluation and necessary treatment.

Therapy started on Monday of the first week and went on for 4.5 weeks. Radiotherapy was performed with daily fractions of 1.8 Gy to the primary and regional lymph nodes. The radiation technique was isocentric, parallel-

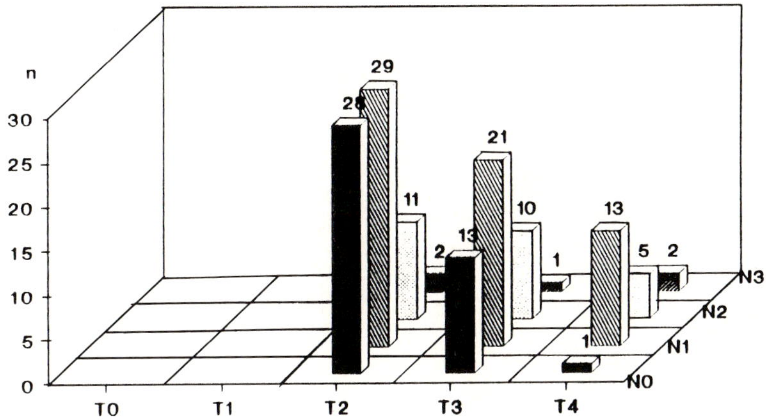

Fig. 1. Clinical tumor classification before therapy (n = 136)

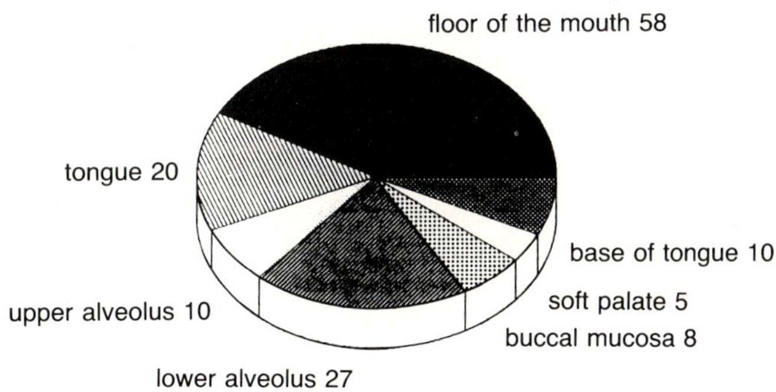

Fig. 2. Distribution of tumor localizations (n = 136; two patients had two localizations)

opposed head and neck fields and an additional ventral field for the caudal cervical and supraclavicular lymph drainage. To guarantee exact positioning for radiation treatment on a day-to-day basis, individually formed head masks were prepared for all patients. Simulation of the radiation fields could then be performed according to tumor site and lymph nodes. Patients were treated with 5 MeV photons of a linear accelerator. The total dose to the tumor and regional lymph chains was 39.6 Gy.

Chemotherapy was given simultaneously on days 1–5 in week 1. One hour before the daily fraction of radiation, patients received 20 mg cisplatin/m^2 body surface area as short-term infusion intravenously with pre- and post-hyperhydration. Two weeks after the end of radiochemotherapy, all patients were restaged. Those with CR or PR underwent surgery, while those with no change or progressive disease continued radiotherapy up to 70.2 Gy to the primary and 56–60 Gy to the lymph nodes combined with a second

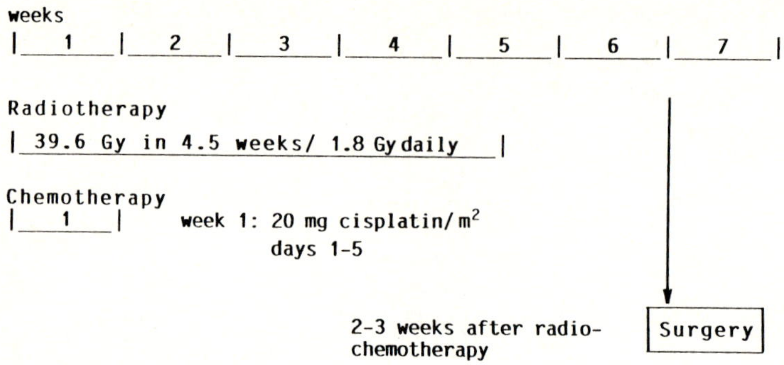

Fig. 3. Treatment Schedule

course of cisplatin (Fig. 3). Surgery of the primary and neck nodes was done according to the guidelines of the German, Austrian, and Swiss Association for Head and Neck Tumors (DÖSAK), as defined in 1982.

Results

After 39.6 Gy radiation therapy and 100 mg cisplatin/m^2, 128 out of 136 patients (94%) could be downstaged (Table 1). A total of 101 out of 136 patients underwent surgery with no further treatment and six of 136 patients received postoperative radiotherapy up to 70.2 Gy with a second course of cisplatin because of tumor in the surgical margins. A total of 22 out of 136 patients were definitively treated with radiochemotherapy up to 70.2 Gy – they had intercurrent diseases or refused surgery. In seven out of 136 cases, therapy was not performed according to the protocol; two of these patients had progressive disease and developed distant metastases during treatment.

The evaluation of recurrence and survival data was done for patients with radiochemotherapy followed by surgery and for those with the full dose of radiochemotherapy (70.2 Gy + 2 × 100 mg cisplatin/m^2). A total of 45 out of 101 patients with radiochemotherapy and surgery clinically showed CR after 39.6 Gy and 100 mg cisplatin/m^2. In 37 of 101 patients, there was no tumor in the surgical specimen; most of these patients initially had T2 cancers. With a median observation time of 38 months for the whole group, the 2-year recurrence rate for the combined treated group (radiochemotherapy and surgery) is 14.9%, for patients with radiochemotherapy only, 56.3%. According to Kaplan and Meier (1958), the survival is also significantly different. After radiochemotherapy and surgery, the 1-year survival rate is 94%, the 2-year survival rate 84%, and the 3-year survival rate 79%. Treated with definitive radiochemotherapy only, 55% survived 1 year, 41% 2 years, and 27% 3 years (Table 2).

Table 1. Classification of tumors according to TNM staging (UICC 1987) (n = 136)

	T0	T1	T2	T3	T4
Before therapy					
N0			28	13	1
N1			29	21	13
N2			11	10	5
N3			2	1	2
After therapy[a]					
N0	45	47	9	1	
N1		20	9		
N2			2	2	1
N3					

[a] Therapy consisted of 39.6 Gy plus 100 mg cisplatin/m^2.

Table 2. Remission and survival

	RT/ChT+OP	Definitive RT/ChT
Patients (n)	101	22
Complete remission (n, %)	98 (97)	15 (68)
Survival (%)		
1 year	94	55
2 years	84	41
3 years	79	27
Local recurrence in 2 years (%)	15	56

RT, radiotherapy; ChT, chemotherapy; OP, surgery.

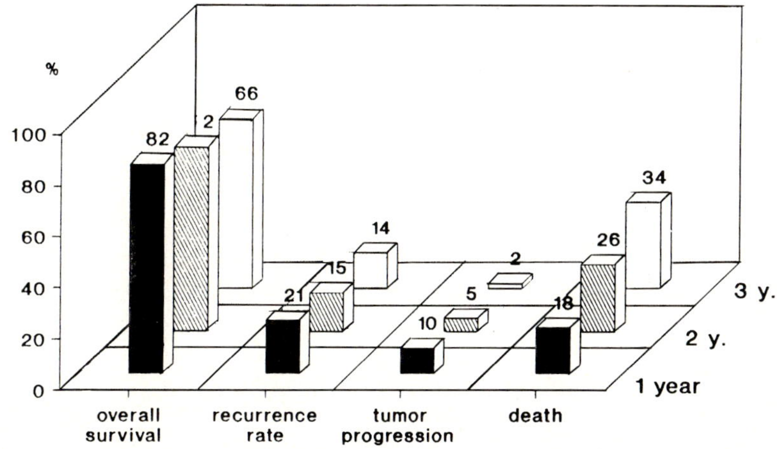

Fig. 4. Follow-up (January 1986–October 1991; n = 136)

The follow-up is shown in Fig. 4. Most failures occurred during the first 2 years after therapy with locoregional recurrent disease. A total of 32% of the patients who failed developed distant metastases, mainly in the lung and bones.

The best response to preoperative radiochemotherapy and the lowest failure rate of 10% was found in patients with a T2 N0–1 carcinoma. There is no difference in remission or survival related to tumor locations. There were tolerable side effects comparable to radiotherapy alone in all patients except one. This 67-year-old man had a heart attack during hyperhydration, probably induced by volume load. There were no radiochemotherapy-related surgical problems or complications and no delay in wound healing.

Discussion

From the early 1980s, many authors have investigated combined radiochemotherapy protocols to improve local control and survival of advanced head and neck carcinomas. With regard to the relatively good prognosis of oral cavity carcinomas compared to other pharyngeal tumor locations, the control rates of large primaries with lymph node metastases are disappointing, as mentioned by Platz et al. (1986). Radiotherapy and simultaneous cisplatin administration in different schedules has proven effective in various clinical trials (Coughlin and Richmond 1985; Haselow et al. 1982; Keizer et al. 1984; Murthy et al. 1985).

The data from 101 patients with advanced oral cavity carcinomas who had preoperative simultaneous radiochemotherapy with cisplatin followed by surgery were evaluated and compared with to 22 patients who received radiochemotherapy up to 70.2 Gy and two courses of cisplatin only. For the combined treated group with surgery, the actuarial 2-year survival rate is 84%, and the local recurrence rate after 2 years is 15%. There is a benefit in survival and local control of about 20% compared to results of historical reference studies with postoperative radiotherapy (Platz et al. 1986). High effectiveness of radiochemotherapy with cisplatin in advanced oral cavity and oropharynx carcinomas was also shown by Zamboglou et al. (1989). He documented more than 70% CR and PR after 40 Gy and 100 mg cisplatin/m^2. The poor results of the small group of patients we treated with radiochemotherapy only may be a negative selection with inoperability due to intercurrent diseases. The CR rate of 68% at the end of therapy is similar to the results of intensive radiochemotherapy studies reported by Duehmke et al. (1988) and Wendt et al. (1989). In these trials, radiation was given in accelerated fractionation, which may be useful in fast repopulating cancers such as head and neck carcinomas, as advocated by Trott and Kummermeh (1985). However, it is important to notice that accelerated radiotherapy produces more severe mucositis as compared to conventional fractionation (Van der Schueren et al. 1983). The treatment schedule we used provoked acceptable acute skin and mucosal reactions with no necessity of a break in radiotherapy or surgery being delayed.

Based on the relatively promising results of this protocol, a randomized trial comparing preoperative radiotherapy and preoperative combined simultaneous radiochemotherapy has been started. As a consequence of the good tolerability of 39.6 Gy, but also a considerably high local recurrence rate of 15% after 2 years, we escalated the radiation dose to 50.4 Gy, given in daily fractions of 1.8 Gy, in both arms of the study. To decrease toxicity of chemotherapy and to avoid hyperhydration related complications carboplatin was substituted for cisplatin. In several trials, the response of advanced head and neck tumors to cisplatin and carboplatin showed no significant difference (Al-Sarraf et al. 1987; Eisenberger et al. 1986; Zamboglou et al. 1988). Chemotherapy is given in the combined arm in week 1 on days 1–5 simultaneously to radiation. One hour before the daily fraction of radiotherapy, patients randomized for combined treatment receive 70 mg carboplatin/m^2 intravenously as short-term infusion without pre- or posthyperhydration. Three to four weeks after radio- or radiochemotherapy, surgery is planned. We hope to achieve more tumor devitalization, especially in gross tumors, with the dose of 50.4 Gy, which may result in a lower local recurrence rate. With randomization, the relative contribution of chemotherapy will be evaluated. For statistically significant results, about 200 patients have to be randomized. First trends will be evaluable in 2 years.

References

Al-Sarraf M, Metch B, Kish J, Enley J, Rinehart JJ, Schuller DE, Coltman CA Jr (1987) Platinum analogs in recurrent and advanced head and neck cancer: a Southwest Oncology Group and Wayne State University study. Cancer Treat Rep 71:723–726

Coughlin CT, Richmond RC (1985) Platinum based combined modality approach for locally advanced head and neck carcinoma. Int J Radiat Oncol Biol Phys 11:915–919

Dewitt L (1987) Combined treatment of radiation and cis-diam-ine-dichloroplatinum (II): a review of experimental and clinical data. Int J Radiat Oncol Biol Phys 13:403–426

DÖSAK (Deutsch-Schweizerisch-Österreichischer Arbeitskreis für Kiefer- und Gesichtschirurgie) (1982) Definitionen zum radichirurgischen Vorgehen bei Plattenepithelkarzinomen der Mundhöhle. Dtsch Z Mund Kiefer Gesichtschir 6:369

Douple EB (1979) Skin radio-sensitization studies using combined cis-diamine-dichloroplatinum (II) and radiation. Int J Radiat Oncol Biol Phys 5:1383–1385

Duehmke E, Geibel T, Golens R (1988) Combined modality treatment of advanced head and neck cancer using low-dose cis-platinum and accelerated fractionation. Strahlenther Onkol 164:11–16

Eisenberger M, Hornedo J, Silva H, Donehower R, Spaulding M, Echo DV (1986) Carboplatin (NSC-241-240): an active platinum analog for the treatment of squamous cell carcinoma of the head and neck. J Clin Oncol 4:1506–1509

Fletcher GH (1980) Textbook of radiotherapy, 3rd edn. Lea and Febinger, Philadelphia

Gefeller D, Renner K, Slomska J (1983) Remissionsbeurteilung einer simultan kombinierten Strahlen-Platintherapie bei progressiven Tumorerkrankungen. Vortrag Deutscher Röntgenkongress, Hannover

Gefeller D, Bendel V, Osterwald L (1987) Low-dose-Platin-Strahlen-sensibilisieru g bei Hals Nasen-Ohren-Tumoren. In: Sauer R, Schwab W (eds) Kombinatioustherapie der Oropharynx und Hypopharynxkarzinane. Urban and Schwarzenberg, Munich

Glanzmann C (1978) Ergebnisse der Radiotherapie des Tosillenkarzinoms bei 161 Patienten. Behandlungszeitraum 1950–1976. Strahlenther Onkol 154:753–757

Haselow RE, Adams GS, Oken MM, Goudsmit A, Lerner HJ, Marsh JC (1982) Simultaneous cis-platinum (DDP) and radiation therapy (RT) for locally advanced unresectable head and neck cancer. Proc Am Soc Clin Oncol 1:201

Jacobs C (1984) The use of chemotherapy in combination with radiotherapy in the treatment of head and neck squamous cancers. In: Wolf GH (ed) Head and neck oncology. Nijhoff, Boston, pp 265–286

Kaplan EL, Meier P (1958) Non parametric estimation from incomplete observations. J Am Stat Assoc 53:457

Keizer HJ, Karim ABMF, Njo KJ, Tiere AH, Snow GB, Vermorken JB, Pindeo HM (1984) Feasibility study on daily administration of cis-diamine-dichloroplatinum (II) in combination with radiotherapy. Radiother Oncol 1:227–234

Kutzner J, Braun E, Mika H (1982) Ergebnisse der Strahlentherapie des Zungenkarzinoms. Strahlenther Onkol 158:470–472

Mendenhall WM, Million RR, Cassisi NJ (1987) Carcinoma of the head and neck. In: Perez CA, Brady LW (eds) Principles and practice of radiation oncology. Lippincott, Philadelphia

Murthy AK, Taylor SG, Showel J, Kramer T, Kiel K, Caldarelli DD, Hutchinson JC, Holinger LD, Witt TR (1985) Improved results with simultaneous chemotherapy and radiation in head and neck cancer. Proc Am Soc Clin Oncol 4:138

Platz H, Fries M, Hudec M (1986) Prognosis of oral cavity carcinomas. Hanser, Munich

Schmitt G, Higi M, Stupp H, Scherer E (1983) Ein neues interdisziplinäres Behandlungskonzept bei fortgeschrittenen Kopf-Hals-Tumoren. Strahlentherapie 159:470–473

Trott KR, Kummermehr J (1985) What is known about tumor proliferation rates to choose between accelerated fractionation or hyperfractionation? Radiother Oncol 3:1–9

UICC (Union Internationale Contre le Cancer) (1987) TNM – Klas-sifikation der malignen Tumoren. Springer, Berlin Heidelberg New York

Van der Schueren E, van de Bogaert W, Ang KK (1983) Radiotherapy with multiple fractions per day. In: Steel GG, Adams GE, Peckham MJ (eds) The biological basis of radiotherapy. Elsevier, Amsterdam

Vikram B, Strong EW, Shah J, Spiro RH (1980) Elevtive postoperative radiation therapy in stage III and IV epidermoid carcinoma of the head and neck. Am J Surg 140:580–584

Wendt TG, Hartenstein RC, Wustrow TPU, Lissner J (1989) Cisplatin, fluorouracil with leucovorin calcium enhancement and synchronous accelerated radiotherapy in the management of locally advanced head and neck cancer: a phase II study. J Clin Oncol 7:471–476

Zamboglou N, Schmitt C, Pape H, Fürst G, Schmitt G (1988) Aspekte der kombinierten Radio-Chemotherapie bei fortgeschrittenen Kopf-Halstumoren. Tumor Diagn Ther 9:35–40

Zamboglou N, Pape H, Schabel T, Wurm R, Bannach G, Fürst G, Schmitt G (1989) Kombinierte Radiotherapie mit Cis- oder Carboplatin bei fortgeschrittenen Kopf-Hals-Tumoren Strahlenther Onkol 165:647–651

Results from DÖSAK Observational Studies

H.-P. Howaldt[1], M. Frenz[2], and H. Pitz[2]

[1] Johann Wolfgang Goethe-University Medical School, Department of Maxillofacial Surgery, Theodor-Stern-Kai 7, 60596 Frankfurt am Main, Germany
[2] Johann Wolfgang Goethe-University Medical School, Center of Medical Informatics, DÖSAK Central Tumor Registry Theodor-Stern-Kai 7, 60596 Frankfurt am Main, Germany

Introduction

In order to gain any valuable information concerning prognostic data of a tumor entity, really good cooperation between many institutions is necessary. By performing standardized documentation and therapy, relevant data can be evaluated once the follow-up of the patients is complete.

As these main assets are well known all over the medical world many cooperative groups such as the Eastern Cooperative group, the European Organization for Research on Treatment of Cancer (EORTC), and the German, Austrian, and Swiss Association for Head and Neck Tumors (DÖSAK) have been established. The main task of the latter group, founded in 1969, is to perform clinical trials and observational studies on tumors of the maxillofacial region (Hausamen 1988). After performing two observational studies and standardizing the documentation, a central tumor registry has been established. This paper presents the work of the DÖSAK group, which consists of more than 80 institutions for maxillofacial surgery in Germany, Austria, and Switzerland.

DÖSAK Retrospective and Prospective Observational Studies

DÖSAK performed two multicenter observational studies. The first was a retrospective one and contained about 1000 patients treated between 1952 and 1972. A consecutive, prospectively designed study was done between 1977 and 1985. Here, around 1500 patients could be followed up successfully. The basis for these two observational studies was a documentation form designed by the Viennese Statisticians' Group. All patients were treated according to the DÖSAK rules concerning radical surgery and the indication for neck dissection, as published by Bier (DÖSAK 1982). As the main result of these two observational studies, a treatment-dependent prognostic index

(TPI) and a more sophisticated computer program for an individual prognosis, called computer-aided individual prognosis (CIP; CIP 1991), was developed by Platz et al. (1986).

Treatment-Dependent Prognostic Index

As mentioned above, the TPI was derived from the retrospective study. Five factors showed significant influence on survival. The factors and their categories are as follows: (1) age of the patient in years ($x \leqslant 50$; $50 < x \leqslant 70$; $70 < x$); (2) tumor size ($x \leqslant 40$ mm; 40 mm $< x$); (3) depth of tumor infiltration ($x \leqslant 5$ mm; 5 mm $< x$); (4) evidence of fixed lymph nodes; and (5) presence of distant metastases.

By combining all possible distinct values of these factors, 48 main groups were generated. Each main group was split up into four subgroups by distinguishing between the combinations of two additional treatment-dependent factors. These are: (1) modalities of treatment (radical surgery alone; nonradical surgery or adjuvant radiotherapy) and (2) therapeutic effect (no evidence of disease; evidence of disease).

For each of the 192 subgroups, a prognostic index was estimated by analyzing the survival data with a multivariate statistical model. The prognostic index was used to compute a survival curve for every subgroup. For every main group, a so-called prognosis sheet was drawn up. It contains the survival rates from 1 to 5 years and a median survival time for all four subgroups. These sheets are part of the book which constitutes the TPI (Platz et al. 1986).

To use the TPI in clinical practice, the physician first has to manually ascertain which TPI subgroup his patient belongs to. Secondly, he has to refer to the book in order to find the corresponding prognosis sheet. This procedure had frequently been used for clinical trials in order to form homogeneous patient groups, but has not been applied to clinical routine.

Computer-Aided Individual Prognosis

To verify the TPI, a prospective study was performed by DÖSAK in which a total of 1485 patients were evaluated. By analyzing the new data, the five pretherapeutic TPI factors age, tumor diameter, tumor infiltration depth, evidence of fixed lymph nodes, and evidence of distant metastasis in general showed the influence expected from the retrospective study. Whereas a better prognosis of lip tumors could not significantly be proven in the retrospective study, the higher number of these tumors in the prospective study leads to a significant difference in prognosis when comparing lip tumors with tumors of the oral cavity and oropharynx.

Furthermore, on the basis of the data from the prospective study, a new prognostic model has been developed. Tumors of the lip are now subject to a separate prognostic model, in which only three factors (sex, age, and tumor infiltration depth) form the basis for calculating the prognosis. For the oral cavity and oropharyx site, separate prognostic models (differing between no evidence of disease and evidence of disease) have been developed. In this interesting model (oral cavity and oropharyx; no evidence of disease), the following factors determine the chances of survival: (a) sex of the patient, (b) age of the patient in years, (c) tumor size in cm, (d) tumor infiltration into adjacent structures ($x \leq 5$ mm; $5 < x$ mm), (e) tumor site by areas (pre- or postcanine; retromolar), (f) evidence of fixed lymph nodes, and (g) treatment modalities (palliative surgery +radiotherapy; radiotherapy; radical surgery ⟨+radiotherapy⟩ ⟨+chemotherapy⟩; curative chemotherapy ⟨+radiotherapy⟩ ⟨+nonradical surgery⟩; nonradical surgery ⟨radiotherapy⟩ ⟨+noncurative chemotherapy⟩). The inclusion criteria for this model are: (a) no palliative surgery, (b) no selective lymph node excision, and (c) no distant metastases.

It is obvious that the large number of possible combinations of these factors makes the model prohibitive for manual usage. For this reason, the prognosis sheets of the TPI have been substituted by a program for personal computers. This program (CIP) has been available since 1991.

Comparison of Survival Within the Retrospective and Prospective Studies

When comparing the prospective and retrospective observational studies of DÖSAK, one is faced with an astonishing result (Fig. 1). The 5-year survival rates of the two samples differ only by about 2.5%, although there are more than 20 years between the observations. Within this period, many new treatment modalities have been added, such as chemotherapy and improvements in radiotherapy as well as in surgery. At every congress on head and neck cancer, many improvements are presented, but it seems that they hardly result in a better chance of survival for patients. On the other hand, this negative conclusion does not completely correspond to reality, as we really do not know whether the two samples of the studies were prognostically equivalent at the beginning of the observation. It is possible that we now operate on more severe cases than in former times.

The Current State of Prognostic Models

Remarkable progress can be seen in establishing multicenter cooperation for observing tumor patients. By developing the TPI and the CIP, the group of Platz, Fries, and Hudec introduced the use of sophisticated and

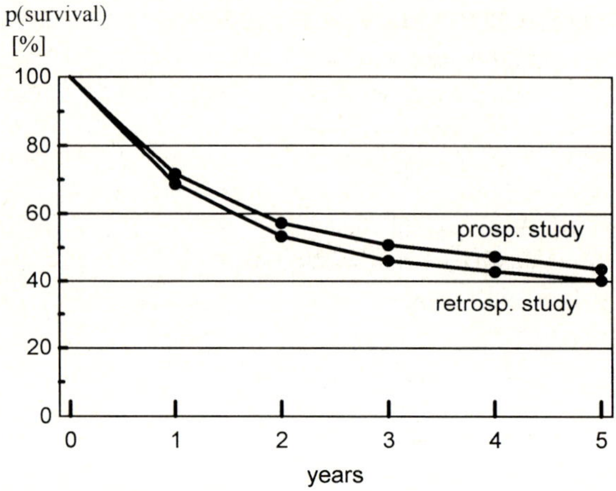

Fig. 1. Survival curves of the retrospective (n = 1022) and prospective (n = 1485) DÖSAK studies (modified according to Platz et al. 1988)

suitable statistical analysis with methods such as the Cox model to our field. Nowadays, the need for these methods is well recognized even by our medical doctors, who are normally not so familiar with statistics, and the progress concerning results is essentially the development of the TPI and the CIP models themselves.

At present, a limitation of this work has to be seen in the design of the documentation forms, which resulted in a limited data quality. Additionally, the lack of a pathology report in the documentation limited the increase in our understanding of a patient's prognosis. The aim of the DÖSAK tumor registry is to collect a higher number of patients with more detailed data and to improve the data quality by supporting on-time documentation, i.e. the patient has to be treated and documented at the same time and, wherever possible, by the same physician.

Standardized Documentation of the Association of German Tumor Centers

After completion of the prospective study, DÖSAK was faced with the need to develop a new documentation standard. By increasing documentation and designing more practical tumor assessment forms, it was possible to establish a widely accepted standard. The aim was to achieve a more detailed observation of the tumors of the maxillofacial region; it should be suitable for all malignancies, though primarily designed for oral cancer.

During the same period, the Association of German Tumor Centers (ADT) started to develop a site-specific documentation standard for all major tumor entities or sites. The DÖSAK group contributed to this effort and developed its new standard in cooperation with the ADT (Howaldt

1987). A set of these forms consists of eight sheets, including patient's admission, diagnosis, therapy, pathology report, follow-up, and termination of study. It was new to include a pathology report in the documentation standard. Its main items are several tumor measurements, the lymph node status according to TNM levels and information concerning grading and extranodal spread of lymph node metastases. In order to gain proper information, the resected specimen with marked areas according to the TNM levels should be sent to the pathologist. The pathohistological findings should be documented directly by the pathologist onto the standardized form. In order to achieve homogeneous usage, some proposals for a standardized documentation, especially for measurement of the tumor thickness, have been published (Howaldt and Herrmann 1989). This documentation has been accepted by all DÖSAK institutions. It forms the basis for the DÖSAK Central Tumor Registry (Howaldt 1992).

The DÖSAK Central Tumor Registry

In 1989, a central tumor registry was established with a grant from the Deutsche Krebshilfe - Dr. Mildred Scheel Stiftung (German Cancer Aid). Its main task is to collect data from all DÖSAK institutions in order to improve knowledge about therapy and prognosis of oral cancer. One main advantage will be achieved by including a standardized pathology report. The aim of the project is to verify previous DÖSAK work, including the TPI and the CIP, and to derive new prognostic factors from the registry's documentation.

Participation

Up to now (April 1992), 56 institutions from three countries have entered almost 5000 patients into the DÖSAK registry. The cumulative number of patients being entered into the registry per quarter shows the constant work of the DÖSAK group (Fig. 2).

Data Quality

The registry itself can only provide methods for improvement of data quality and on-time documentation. For every patient, an overview containing brief information concerning the most important tumor and treatment items is printed. It has proved to be a useful tool in the hospital during patient's treatment and follow-up. In addition, it allows the doctor to detect documentation errors. A large variety of plausibility programs have been developed to detect missing items, logical errors, and rare combinations of

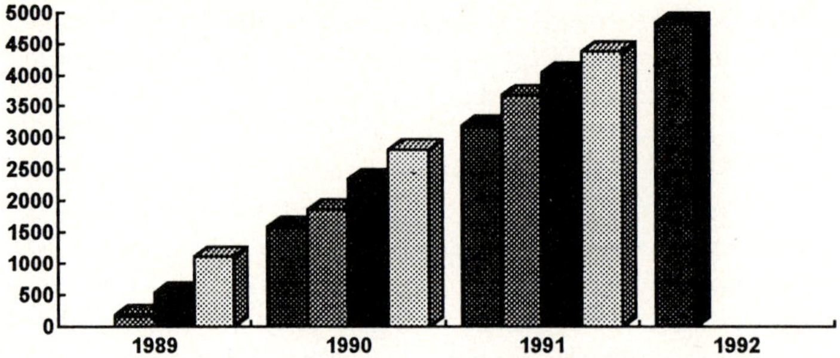

Fig. 2. Cumulative number of patients in the registry's data base

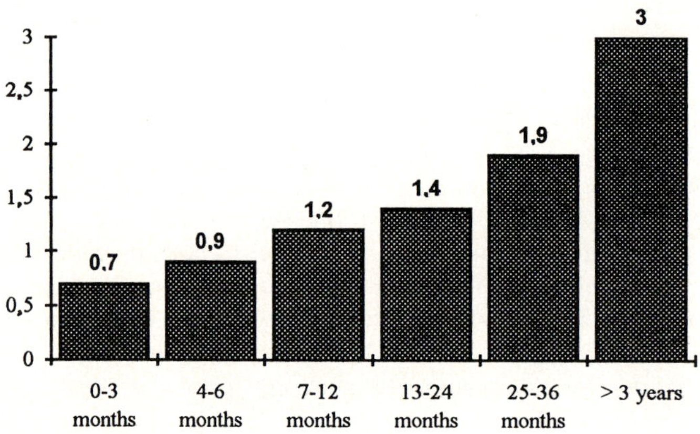

Fig. 3. Relation between data quality measured in avarage number of documentation errors within plausibility control (*y-axis*) and time from diagnosis to entering the data (*x-axis*)

findings. Furthermore, doctor's letters can be provided to support an on-time documentation.

It is quite interesting to demonstrate a direct relation between data quality measured by the average number of documentation errors, and the delay between documentation and entering in the registry. The faster the documentation forms reach the registry, the better the data quality is (Fig. 3).

Tumor Entities

Within the registry's data base, there are 3148 cases of primary squamous cell carcinomas of the oral cavity, including lips and oropharynx. The main

Table 1. Frequency of tumor entities in the Central Tumor Registry

Tumor entity	No. of patients
Squamous cell carcinomas of the oral cavity and oropharynx	3148
Squamous cell carcinomas of the skin	160
Basal cell carcinomas	157
Salivary gland tumors	90
Malignant melanomas	90
Unknown primaries	64
Other squamous cell carcinomas	63
Adenoid cystic carcinomas	62
Paranasal sinus tumors	57

interest of the registry is focused on this entity. The remaining part of the sample consists of adenoid cystic carcinomas, salivary gland tumors, melanomas, skin cancer, and various other more or less rare entities which are treated by maxillofacial surgeons. Table 1 shows the frequencies of the major tumor entities.

Each individual institution has too few cases to derive certain scientific information from these cases; a multicenter cooperation is, therefore, indispensible. Our former results show that only small steps in the progress of cancer treatment regarding survival have been made in the past few decades. In order to detect relatively small improvements, we need large numbers of homogeneously documented cases.

Follow-Up

The follow-up service of the registry is very important in order to obtain early and complete information about recurrence and survival of the patients, which is the most important criteria for the success of treatment. Other criteria such as quality of life are not as objective as lifetime and are currently not subject to our investigations.

After 3 years of work, the DÖSAK registry's data are still at a relatively early stage, which is why it is not yet possible to show definite results concerning prognostic factors or survival rates. In other words, the percentage of censored values concerning survival is too high to be able to produce survival curves which are comparable to other observational studies already finished.

Figure 4 presents the actual survival data of all primary cases of squamous cell carcinomas of the oral cavity and oropharynx (Frenz et al. 1992). The percentage of censored observations in the data is 78%.

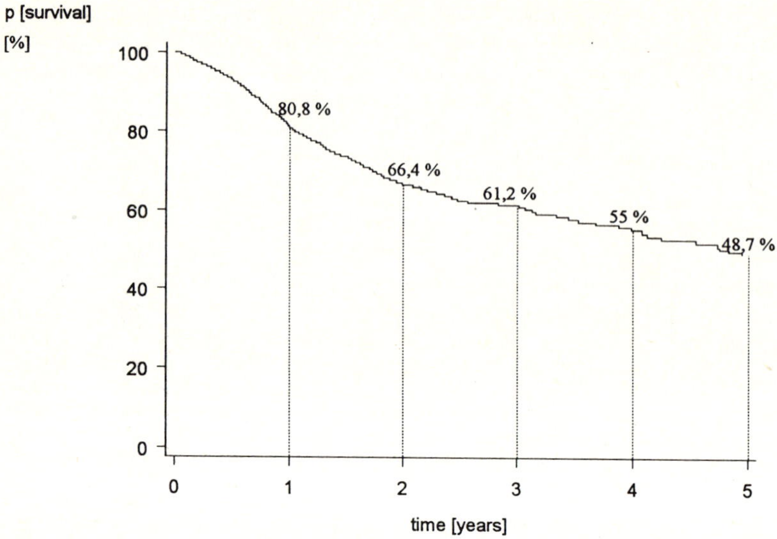

Fig. 4. Kaplan-Meier survival curve for primary squamous cell carcinomas of the oral cavity and oropharynx (n = 3148)

Analysis of Patients Not Operated

Although the following data are only preliminary, it is interesting to look at the survival curves of all patients with primary squamous cell carcinomas of the oral cavity and oropharynx who have not been operated, amounting to 13%. Due to the quite poor prognosis of this group, it is possible to do reliable survival analysis even after a follow-up period of only 3 years.

Out of 412 patients, about one third had received radiotherapy alone, one third was treated by radiotherapy and chemotherapy, and one third received only chemotherapy or no treatment at all. When comparing the survival curves of the radiotherapy and radiochemotherapy group, an effect that has been frequently reported before can be seen. In the group treated with radiotherapy and chemotherapy, the survival is slightly prolonged, although the 5-year survival rate is not improved (Fig. 5).

Conclusions

We have to recognize that with our present tools against oral cancer, we will only be able to achieve small and stepwise improvements of survival. It is of common interest which factors are responsible for the outcome of treatment of our patients. We must acknowledge the fact that our present therapy modalities do not have the great effect that many surgeons believe they do.

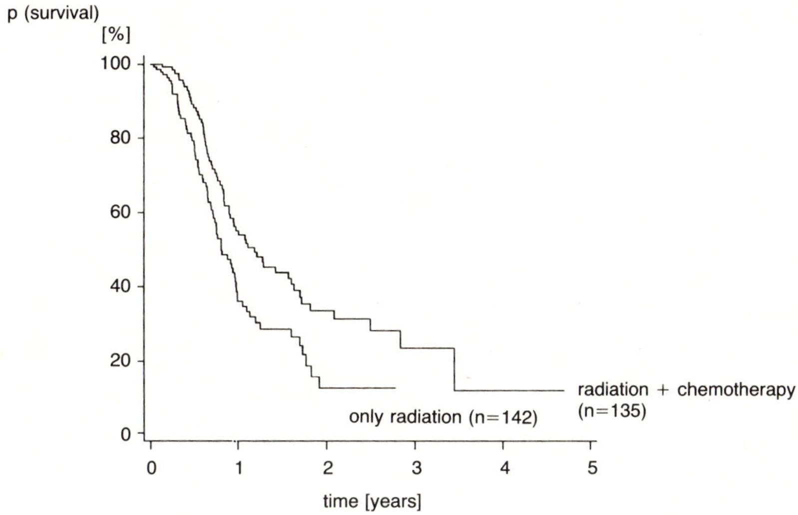

Fig. 5. Survival curves for patients with radiotherapy alone compared to radiotherapy-chemotherapy combination

One consequence of this fact should be that we have to pay more attention to the quality of life of our patients. The prognostic factors being investigated in the work of the present registry will be important for our treatment planning; we hope to have a better idea which of our patients require a more aggressive treatment and in which cases it can be avoided. In addition, the knowledge of as many prognostic factors as possible is needed for our forthcoming scientific work in randomized trials in order to allow proper interpretation of our results.

Acknowledgements. The DÖSAK tumor registry described in this paper is supported by the Deutsche Krebshilfe - Dr. Mildred Scheel Stiftung Bonn.

References

CIP (1991) Computerunterstützte individuelle Prognosestellung für Plattenepithelkarzinome der Lippen, der Mundhöhle und des Oropharynx. Handbuch. Data Technology, Vienna

DÖSAK (1982) Definitionen zum radikalchirurgischen Vorgehen bei Plattenepithelcarzinomen der Mundhöhle. Dtsch Z Mund Kiefer Gesichtschir 6:369–372

Frenz M, Howaldt HP, Pitz H (1992) 3. Projektbericht. Zentrales Tumorregister des DÖSAK. Frankfurt University Hospital

Hausamen JE (1988) Tasks and objectives of the German Austrian Swiss working group on tumors in the maxillo-facial region (DÖSAK). Int J Oral Maxillofac Surg 17:264–266

Howaldt HP (1987) Die Dokumentation mit dem ADT-Tumorbogen für Malignome des Mundes, der Kiefer und des Gesichts. Dtsch Z Mund Kiefer Gesichtschir 11:417–427

Howaldt HP (1992) Tumor-Dokumentation im Mund-Kiefer-Gesichtsbereich. Aufbau und Ergebnisse als Grundlage für ein überregionales Register. Hanser, Munich

Howaldt HP, Herrmann G (1989) Standardisierte pathoanatomische Befunddokumentation auf den ADT-Tumorbögen für Malignome des Mundes, der Kiefer und des Gesichts. Pathologe 10:364–368

Platz H, Fries R, Hudec M (1986) Prognoses of oral cavity carcinomas. Results of a multicentric retrospective observational study. Hanser, Munich

Platz H, Fries R, Hudec M (1988) Einführung in die "Prospektive DÖSAK-Studie über Plattenepithelkarzinome der Lippen, der Mundhöhle und des Oropharynx." Dtsch Z Mund Kiefer Gesichtschir 12:293–302

Current Trends in Therapeutic Research

H. Bier

Department of Otorhinolaryngology/Head and Neck Surgery, Heinrich-Heine-Universität, Moorenstrasse 5, 40225 Düsseldorf, Germany

Introduction

In general, the treatment of squamous cell carcinoma of the oral cavity and the oropharynx is confined to the established measures surgery, radiotherapy, and chemotherapy. Three treatment strategies currently under preclinical and clinical investigation that are of potential value to complement and hopefully to improve our therapeutic efforts are: prevention of disease, immunotherapy, and circumvention of drug resistance.

Prevention of Disease

Extensive experiments in animal models have identified two major steps in the multifactorial development of cancer: (1) initiation and (2) promotion. Since initiation involves genotypic alteration, it is generally considered as irreversible. Promotion is characterized by several phenotypic changes, including cellular hyperplasia, nuclear polymorphism, and disordered or absent maturation. Based on current knowledge of the carcinogenesis process, at least three types of prevention can be defined: (1) primary prevention by avoiding or removing the sources of known carcinogens; however, with regard to head and neck cancer, social modification of smoking and alcohol habits seems unlikely; (2) secondary prevention by modulation of the interaction between active agents and host tissue on different levels of the multistep carcinogenesis process, e.g., interference with carcinogen metabolism, activation or support of detoxication pathways, and DNA repair mechanisms; (3) tertiary prevention by suppression or reversal of already established preneoplastic lesions. The latter type of prevention gains particular importance in head and neck cancer, as the phenomenon of "field cancerization" is a key feature of the upper aero-digestive tract: multiple foci of intraepithelial neoplasia progressing concurrently to form multiple, usually metachronous primary carcinomas (de Vries, this volume).

Of the several compounds that have been identified as antipromotor or progressing blocking agents, vitamin A analogs are certainly the best investigated (Lippman and Hong 1992). Retinoids exert a hormone-like control of proliferation and differentiation in essentially all epithelia that are target sites for the development of carcinoma. So far, two major aspects of the interaction of retinoids and epithelial cells have been characterized in experimental models: (1) suppression of phenotypic transformation initiated by a variety of carcinogens and (2) inhibition of malignant proliferation, predominantly through induction of differentiation (Sporn et al. 1992).

Two receptor families comprising at least six distinct retinoid receptors have now been identified, both of which have different preferred ligands (Giguere et al. 1987; Petkovich et al. 1987). These receptors are believed to be involved in the modulation of growth-controlling signals. Furthermore, the effect of retinoids appears to be mediated by increased synthesis of the regulatory peptide-transforming growth factor beta (TGF-β). TGF-β has pleiotropic effects on cell growth and differentiation and most likely acts as a negative autocrine factor in the control of epithelial cell proliferation (Moses 1992). In addition, retinoids are able to stimulate both humoral and cellular immunity. On the one hand, these multiple biologic effects of retinoids give us a notion of the sophisticated network of cell growth regulation. On the other hand, the molecular characterization of chemoprevention mechanisms will enable us to develop new strategies for disease prevention.

The clinical introduction of preventive agents for cancer is divided into three phases: (1) feasibility studies, (2) limited intervention trials, and (3) extended intervention trials (Castonguay 1992). With regard to the use of retinoids in head and neck cancer patients, encouraging first results were reported by Hong et al. (1990). However, we have to realize that the incidence of second primary cancers in the placebo arm of this particular study in unusually high (Snow 1991). The results of the EUROSCAN trial using retinyl palmitate and *N*-acetyl-L-cysteine are eagerly awaited (de Vries et al. 1991), and another multicenter chemoprevention trial with low-dose 13-*cis* retinoic acid in early stage head and neck cancer was initiated in the United States last year (Lippmon and Hong 1992). The development of biomarkers which correlate with the regression of intraepithelial neoplasia is highly desirable, because they can provide modulatable intermediate end points in chemoprevention trials, thus avoiding presently required long-term, large-population studies (Lee et al. 1992; Tockmann et al. 1992).

Immunotherapy

Our current understanding of tumor immunology implies that effective immunotherapy might be possible by: (1) enhancement of tumor antigenicity/

immunogenicity, (2) stimulation/support of the host's specific/nonspecific immune reactions, and (3) inhibition of immune suppression (de Vita et al. 1991). Until today, the majority of immunotherapeutic approaches in human malignancies have been disappointing. However, in recent years concepts of tumor immunology have undergone further development, and we have gained better insight into biological interactions between the tumor and its host (Wolf 1984; den Otter and Ruitenberg 1987; Metzgar and Mitchel 1988; de Vita et al. 1991 Vlock 1991).

In general, lymphocytes are the most prominent cellular component of inflammatory infiltrates in head and neck carcinomas, but as yet the significance of this lymphocytic reaction remains controversial. More recent investigations have analyzed phenotype and function of tumor-infiltrating lymphocytes (TIL) in head and neck carcinomas (Rabin et al. 1984; Miescher et al. 1986; Wolf et al. 1986; Heo et al. 1987; Mickel et al. 1988; Snyderman et al. 1989). T lymphocytes make up the major TIL component, and compared to autologous peripheral blood lymphocytes, there is a significant increase in activated T cells, as judged by the expression of human leukocyte DR (HLA-DR) antigens and interleukin-2 (IL-2) receptors (Whiteside et al. 1989). However, the proportion of natural killer NK cells is decreased. Unfortunately, freshly isolated TIL were found to be poor in vitro effectors of antitumor cytotoxicity, and they exhibited profound unresponsiveness to different activating agents (Whiteside et al. 1988). These refractory responses of TILs and the failure to outgrow tumor-specific T lymphocytes (CTL) from TIL preparations has led to considerable disappointment, particularly because studies in numerous murine models and, for example, human malignant melanoma (de Vries and Spits 1984; Anichini et al. 1986), yielded undisputed evidence for the existence of specific CTLs in tumors (Whiteside et al. 1989), although Cozzolino et al. (1987) have been able to isolate T lymphocytes from tumor-invaded lymph nodes that can be induced to proliferate specifically in response to autologous tumor cells. This autologous in vitro reactivity required supplementation of IL-2 and removal of a distinct suppressor T cell population. Such functional in vitro studies are very important for our understanding of the multifactorial tumor–host relationship, but, unfortunately, squamous cell head and neck carcinomas are troublesome candidates for TIL/tumor cell preparations. Considerable information on the functional capabilities of TILs should be expected from the application of in situ hybridization techniques.

The existence of cytokines has been recognized for many years, but before the 1980s research was progressing slowly because they were only available in minute quantities, and they often contained impurities which confused results. Today, the use of recombinant DNA technology enables us to generate high expression of human protein in simple organisms, thereby providing us with large amounts of defined cytokines. The particular ability of IL-2 to activate numerous immune functions on the T, B, and NK cell and macrophage level that are capable of mediating tumor cell eradication has led to considerable interest in IL-2-based immunotherapy (de

Vita et al. 1991). Besides the systemic administration of high-dose IL-2 either alone or in combination with extracorporally expanded lymphokine-activated killer (LAK) cells or TILs, promising approaches to local and/or regional low-dose IL-2 have been developed in murine tumor models (Forni et al. 1985; Bubenik and Indrova 1987). In particular, intralesional IL-2 treatment has proved to be successful in the strain 2 guinea pig/line 10 hepatocarcinoma model (Mattijssen et al. 1992), which to some extent is considered to be of paradigmatic value for head and neck cancer (Bier et al. 1989). Furthermore, intratumoral IL-2 therapy was able to cure cows suffering from squamous cell carcinoma of the eyelid (Rutten et al. 1989). Cortesina's group in Turin introduced regional low-dose IL-2 treatment in relapsed head and neck cancer patients and achieved objective remissions in six of ten patients (1988). However, other groups have not been able to confirm these encouraging results with identical or modified protocols so far (Mattijssen et al. 1991). Since the patients were heavily pretreated or suffered from considerable tumor burden, we have to recognize the limitations of immunotherapy in such a setting. Therefore, a prospective randomized trial on inductive and adjuvant regional low-dose IL-2 therapy versus conventional treatment alone in patients with advanced, but operable, squamous cell carcinoma of the oral cavity and oropharynx has been initiated.

Another promising aspect of tumor immunology that deserves to be mentioned is the development of monoclonal antibodies (mab) directed against tumor-associated structures. There are numerous potential applications of mabs both in cancer diagnosis, e.g., nuclear scanning/detection with radiolabeled mabs, immunopathology, and in therapy, e.g., primary antibody-dependent cell-mediated (ADCC)/complement-mediated cytotoxicity, conjugated mabs (drugs, toxins, radio-nuclides), or modulation of growth factor receptors. Concerning squamous cell carcinoma of the head and neck, clinically relevant mabs may be K 984 (Schrijvers et al. 1992), E 48 (van Dongen et al. 1992), and the anti epidermal growth factor receptor (EGF-R) mab EMD 55900.

Drug Resistance

The phenomenon of drug resistance is characterized by two well-known clinical observations: either the tumor is primarily unresponsive to chemotherapy, manifested by progressive disease despite initial treatment, or chemotherapy is able to produce dramatic and sometimes complete tumor regressions but, unfortunately, the duration of response is limited to a few months and further chemotherapy is inefficient due to the over-growth of drug-resistant tumor cell subsets in terms of secondary resistance. There are many biological events that can result in tumor resistance to chemotherapy, and in most instances it is probable that the etiology of clinically operational resistance is multifactorial (Chabner 1986; Borst 1991).

One of the most active antineoplastic agents in head and neck cancer is cisplatin (Ganzer et al. 1987). DNA is considered to be the target molecule, and intrastrand cross-links between neighboring guanine bases appear to be the most prevalent type of aduct formation. Three main mechanisms are held responsible for the development of tumor resistance to cisplatin: (1) cisplatin enters the cell by passive diffusion as well as by way of an energy-dependent mechanism; decreased drug uptake into tumor cells has been described for resistant subpopulations (Andrews et al. 1988; Kraker and Moore 1988); (2) the portion of DNA reticulated by cisplatin aducts can be removed and replaced by repair enzymes; increased DNA repair capacity is another reason for the development of drug resistance (Sekiya et al. 1989; Eastman et al. 1988); and (3) the electrophilic cisplatin hydrolysates may be intercepted by nucleophilic compounds before they can react with the critical target DNA; this increased drug inactivation is effected most often by sulfhydryls (Teicher et al. 1987; Sekija et al. 1989; Carmichael et al. 1988). In order to elaborate strategies to overcome drug resistance, in vitro and in vivo models with characterized mechanisms of resistance were established (Teicher et al. 1987). We have introduced a largely defined model of cisplatin resistance in the human squamous carcinoma cell line HLac 79 (Bier et al. 1990). The recloned maternal line ML was divided into four sublines, which were exposed to successively increased, but different, cisplatin concentrations during parallel propagation. The respective dose–response curves as determined by the tetrazolium salt based MTT assay revealed resistance factors ranging from 2.7 to 6.4. The most prominent feature of the resistant sublines were alterations of glutathione metabolism. Three sublines showed significantly elevated intracellular glutathione levels, and in two sublines we found an accompanying increase of the enzyme glutathione-S-transferase to be responsible for the detoxifying conjugation of numerous metabolites and compounds to glutathione.

Glutathione depletion by the synthetic amino acid buthionine sulfoximine (BSO), a specific inhibitor of the enzyme γ-glutamylcysteine synthetase, led to marked reversal of cisplatin resistance in vitro. After subcutaneous transplantation of HLac 79 tumor cells in nude mice, we observed a significant prolongation of survival time for those animals that underwent combined BSO and cisplatin therapy as compared to animals treated with cisplatin alone (Bier 1991). According to recently introduced phase I trials, glutathione reductions of 60%–70% can be achieved in cancer patients (Bailey et al. 1992). Forthcoming studies will have to investigate the potential of BSO to circumvent resistance in patients with drug refractory disease.

Conclusion

The topic of the present paper could easily fill an extra volume (Snow and Clark 1992), and therefore only three aspects of current trends in therapeutic research are addressed in this chapter. Recent advances in the understanding of cancer biology and the availability of new biotechnologies give reason for the optimistic impression that we are perhaps at the end of the beginning of the search for more successful treatment strategies for our cancer patients.

References

Andrews PA, Mann SC, Velury S, Howell SB (1988) Cisplatin uptake mediated cisplatin resistance in human ovarian carcinoma cells. In: Nicolini M (ed) Platinum and other metal coordination compounds in cancer chemotherapy. Nijhoff, Boston, pp 248–254

Anichini A, Fossati G, Parmiani G (1986) Heterogeneity of clones from a human metastatic melanoma detected by autologous cytotoxic T lymphocyte clones. J Exp Med 163:215–223

Bailey H, Mulcahy RT, Iisch KD, Gipp J, Pomplum M, Arzoomanian RZ, Alberti D, Feierabend C, Spriggs D (1992) Glutathione levels and γ-glutamyl-cysteine synthase activity in patients undergoing phase I treatment with L-buthionine sulfoximine and melphalan. Proc Am Assoc Cancer Res 33:479

Bier H (1991) Circumvention of drug resistance in cisplatin-resistant sublines of the human squamous carcinoma cell line HLac 79 in vitro and in vivo. Acta Otolaryngol 111:797–806

Bier H, Armonat G, Bier J, Schirrmacher V, Ganzer U (1989) Postoperative active-specific immunotherapy of lymph node micrometastasis in a guinea pig tumor model. ORL 51:197–205

Bier H, Bergler W, Mikisch G, Wesch H, Ganzer U (1990) Establishment and characterization of cisplatin-resistant sublines of the human squamous carcinoma cell line HLac 79. Acta Otolaryngol 110:466–473

Borst P (1991) Genetic mechanisms of drug resistance. Rev Oncol 4:87–105

Bubenik J, Indrova M (1987) Cancer immunotherapy using local inter-leukin-2 administration. Immunol Lett 16:305–310

Carmichael I, Mitchell JB, Friedmann N, Gazdar AF, Russo A (1988) Glutathione and related enzyme activity in human lung cell lines. Br J Cancer 58:437–440

Castonguay A (1992) Methods and strategies in lung cancer control. Cancer Res [Suppl] 52:2641s–2651s

Chabner BA (1986) Karnofsky memorial lecture: the oncologic end game. J Clin Oncol 4:625–638

Cortesina G, de Stefani A, Giovarelli M, Barioglio MG, Cavallo GP, Jemma C, Forni G (1988) Treatment of recurrent squamous cell carcinoma of the head and neck with low doses of interleukin-2 injected perilymphatically. Cancer 62:2482–2485

Cozzolino F, Torcia M, Carossino AM, Giordani R, Selli C, Talini G, Reali E, Novelli A, Pistoia V, Ferrarini M (1987) Characterization of cells from invaded lymph nodes in patients with solid tumors. J Exp Med 166:303–318

Den Otter W, Ruitenberg EJ (1987) Tumor immunology. Mechanisms, diagnosis, therapy. Elsevier, Amsterdam

De Vita VT, Hellman S, Rosenberg SA (1991) Biologic therapy of cancer. Lippincott, Philadelphia

De Vries JE, Spits H (1984) Cloned human cytotoxic T lymphocyte (CTL) lines reactive with autologous melanoma cells: I. In vitro generation, isolation, and analysis to phenotype and specificity. J Immunol 132:510–518

De Vries N, van Zandwijk N, Pastorino U (1991) The Euroscan study. Br J Cancer 64:985–989

Eastman A, Schulte N, Sheibani N, Sorensen CM (1988) Mechanisms of resistance to platinum drugs. In: Nicolini M (ed) Platinum and other metal coordination compounds in cancer chemotherapy. Nijhoff, Boston, pp 178–196

Forni G, Giovarelli M, Santoni A (1985) Lymphokine-activated tumor inhibition in vivo. The local administration of interleukin-2 triggers nonreactive lymphocytes from tumorbearing mice to inhibit tumor growth. J Immunol 134:1305–1311

Ganzer U, Bier H, Bachert C (1987) Kritische Anmerkungen zur Chemotherapie bösartiger Kopf- und Halsgeschwülste. Laryngol Rhinol Otol 66:200–204

Giguere V, Ong ES, Segui P, Evans RM (1987) Identification of a receptor for the morphogen retinoic acid. Nature 330:624–629

Glick AB, Mc Cune BK, Abdulkarem N, Flanders KC, Lumadue JA, Smith JM, Sporn MB (1991) Complex regulation of TGF-β expression by retinoic acid in the vitamin A-deficient rat. Development 111:1081–1086

Heo DS, Whiteside TL, Johnson JT, Chen K, Barnes EL, Herberman RB (1987) Long term interleukin-2 dependent growth and cytotoxic activity of tumor infiltrating lymphocytes from human squamous cell carcinomas of the head and neck. Cancer Res 47:6353–6362

Hong WK, Lippman SM, Itri LM, Karp DD, Lee JS, Byers RM, Schantz SP, Kramer AM, Lotan R, Peters LJ, Dimery IW, Brown BW, Goepfert H (1990) Prevention of second primary tumors with isoretinoin in squamous cell carcinoma of the head and neck. N Engl J Med 323:795–801

Kliewer SA, Umesono K, Mangelsdorf DJ, Evans RM (1992) Retinoid X receptor interacts with nuclear receptors in retinoic acid, thyroid hormone and vitamin D3 signalling. Nature 355:446–449

Kraker AJ, Moore CW (1988) Accumulation of cis-diamminedichloro-platinum (II) and platinum analogues by platinum-resistant murine leukemia cells in vitro. Cancer Res 48:9–13

Lee JS, Lippman SM, Hong WK, Ro JY, Kim SY, Lotan R, Mittelman WN (1992) Determination of biomarkers for intermediate endpoints in chemoprevention trials. Cancer Res [Suppl] 52:2707s–2710s

Lippman SM, Hong WK (1992) Differentiation agents: a future direction for the management of upper aerodigestive tract squamous cell carcinoma. In: Snow GB, Clark JR (eds) Multimodality therapy for head and neck cancer. Thieme, Stuttgart, pp 160–181

Mattijssen V, De Mulder PH, Schornagel JM, Verweij J, Van den Brock P, Galazka A, Roy S, Ruiter DJ (1991) Clinical and immunopathological results of a phase II study of perilymphatically injected recombinant interleukin-2 in locally far advanced, nonpretreated head and neck squamous cell carcinoma. J Immunother 10:63–68

Mattijssen V, Balemans LTM, Steerenberg PA, De Mulder PHM (1992) Polyethylene glycol modified interleukin-2 superior to recombinant interleukin-2 in locoregional treatment of the line 10 tumor in guinea pigs. J Immunother (in press)

Metzgar RS, Mitchell MS (1988) Human tumor antigens and specific tumor therapy. Liss, New York

Mickel RA, Kessler DJ, Taylor JMG, Lichtenstein A (1988) Natural killer cell cytotoxicity in the peripheral blood, cervical lymph nodes, and tumor of head and neck cancer patients. Cancer Res 48:5017–5022

Miescher S, Whiteside TL, Carrel S, von Fliedner V (1986) Functional properties of tumor infiltrating and blood lymphocytes in patients with solid tumors: effect of tumor cells and their supernatents on proliferative responses of lymphocytes. J Immunol 136:1899–1907

Moses HL (1992) Transforming growth factors and cancer: new insights. Proc Am Assoc Cancer Res 33:560

Mueller BM, Romerdahl CA, Trent JM, Reisfeld RA (1991) Suppression of spontaneous melanoma metastasis in scid mice with an antibody to the epidermal growth factor receptor. Cancer Res 51:2193–2198

Petkovich M, Brand NJ, Krust A, Chambon P (1987) A human retinoic acid receptor which belongs to the family of nuclear receptors. Nature 330:444–450

Rabin BS, Johnson J, Claassen D (1984) Identification of subsets of lymphocytes infiltrating head and neck tumor tissue: a preliminary report. Laryngoscope 94:688–690

Rutten VP, Klein WR, de Jong WA, Misdorp W, den Otter W, Steerenberg PA, De Jong WH, Ruitenberg EJ (1989) Local interleukin-2 therapy in bovine ocular squamous cell carcinoma. Cancer Immunol Immunother 30:165–169

Schrijvers AHGJ, Gerretsen M, van Walsum M, Braakhuis BJM, Quak JJ, Snow GB, van Dongen GAMS (1992) Potential for targeting head and neck squamous cell carcinoma with monoclonal antibody K984. Cancer Immunol Immunother 34:252–258

Sekiya S, Oosaki T, Andoh S, Suzuki N, Akaboshi M, Takamizawa M (1989) Mechanisms of resistance to cis-diamminedichloroplatinum (II) in a rat ovarian carcinoma cell line. Eur J Cancer 25:429–437

Snow GB (1991) Head and neck: editorial overview. Curr Opin Oncol 3:497–499

Snow GB, Clark JR (1992) Multimodality therapy for head and neck cancer. Thieme, Stuttgart

Synderman CH, Heo DS, Chenk (1989) T-cell markers in tumor-infiltrating lymphocytes of head and neck cancer. Head Neck 11:331–337

Sporn MB, Roberts AB, Wakefield LM (1992) Molecular and cellular basis for the use of retinoids in chemorpevention. Proc Am Assoc Cancer Res 33:565–566

Teicher BA, Holden SA, Kelley MJ, Shea TC, Cucchi CA, Rosowsky A, Henner WD, Frei E (1987) Characterization of a human squamous carcinoma cell line resistant to cis-diamminedichloroplatinum (II). Cancer Res 47:388–393

Tockman MS, Gupta PK, Pressman NJ, Mulshine JL (1992) Considerations in bringing a cancer biomarker to clinical application. Cancer Res [Suppl] 52:2711s–2718s

Van der Bruggen P, Traversari C, Chomez P, Lurquin C, de Plaen E, van den Eynde B, Knuth A, Boon T (1991) A gene encoding an antigen recognized by cytolytic T lympocytes on a human melanoma. Science 254:1643–1647

Van Dongen GAMS, Leverstein H, Roos JC, Quak JJ, van den Brekel MWM, Van Lingen A, Martens HJM, Castelijns JA, Visser GWM, Meijer CJLM, Teule GJJ, Snow GB (1992) Radioimmunoscintigraphy of head and neck cancer using 99 Tc-labeled monoclonal antibody E48 F(ab')2. Cancer Res 52:2569–2574

Vlock DR (1991) Immunobiologic aspects of head and neck cancer. Hematol Oncol Clin North Am 5:797–820

Whiteside TL, Heo DS, Takagi S, Johnson JT, Iwatsuki S, Herberman RB (1988) Cytolytic antitumor effector cells in long term cultures of human tumor infiltrating lymphocytes in recombinant interleukin-2. Cancer Immunol Immunother 26:1–10

Whiteside TL, Heo DS, Takagi S, Herbermann RB (1989) Tumor-infiltrating lymphocytes from human solid tumors: antigen-specific killer T lymphocytes of activated natural killer lymphocytes. In: Stevenson HC (ed) Adoptive cellular immunotherapy of cancer. Dekker, New York, pp 139–157

Wolf GT (1984) Head and neck oncology. Nijhoff, Boston

Wolf GT, Hudson JL, Peterson KA, Miller HL, Mc Clatchey KD (1986) Lymphocyte subpopulations in infiltrations of squamous carcinomas of the head and neck: correlations with extent of tumor and prognosis. Otolaryngol Head Neck Surg 95:142–151

The Radiobiology, Treatment, and Prevention of Osteoradionecrosis of the Mandible

E.R. Carlson

Henry Ford Hospital, Department of Surgery, Division of Oral and Maxillofacial Surgery, 2799 West Grand Boulevard, Detroit, Michigan 48202-2689, USA

Introduction

Osteoradionecrosis of the mandible is neither a recently described disease nor a disease limited to the maxillofacial skeleton. Phemister (1926) and Ewing (1926) reported cases of radium necrosis of bone and radiation osteitis, respectively. Furthermore, osteoradionecrosis has been reported in a variety of anatomic sites including the pelvis, femoral head, sternum, and clavicle. Osteoradionecrosis of the mandible, as a debilitating complication of cancericidal irradiation, was not reported with any frequency until the 1950s, when irradiation of oral malignancies became a well-established practice. Since that time, it has become evident that because of the increasing incidence of malignancies of the head and neck, the effectiveness of irradiation in these cancers, the presence of teeth in the jaws, and the functional and cosmetic importance of the mandible, osteoradionecrosis is not only most common in this area, but also tremendously impacts on the patient's quality of life. Numerous publications have followed related to the broad spectrum of presentations of osteoradionecrosis of the mandible, as well as speculation as to the etiology of the disease (Happonen et al. 1983; Obwegeser and Sailer 1978). Indeed, this author's experience includes cases of osteoradionecrosis of the mandible presenting as painless, intraoral areas of exposed mandible, all the way to painful pathologic fractures of the mandible with large orocutaneous fistulae and significant loss of surrounding soft tissue (Figs. 1, 2). As such, the general working, clinical definition of osteoradionecrosis is any exposed bone in a field of irradiation which has failed to heal for at least 6 months.

Perhaps the most equivocal and previously poorly understood aspect of osteoradionecrosis is its etiology. In 1970, Meyer defined a pathogenic sequence of radiation, trauma, and infection responsible for osteoradionecrosis of the mandible. Titterington (1971) subsequently described osteoradionecrosis as a radiation-induced osteomyelitis. It was believed during the

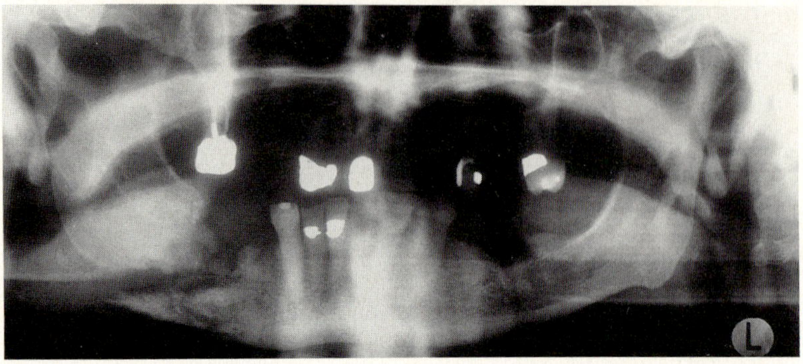

Fig. 1. Panoramic radiograph demonstrating pathologic fracture associated with osteoradionecrosis of the mandible. This fracture occurred approximately 2 months after tooth extraction and 5 years after tumoricidal radiotherapy. Patients with pathologic fractures immediately enter stage 3 protocol

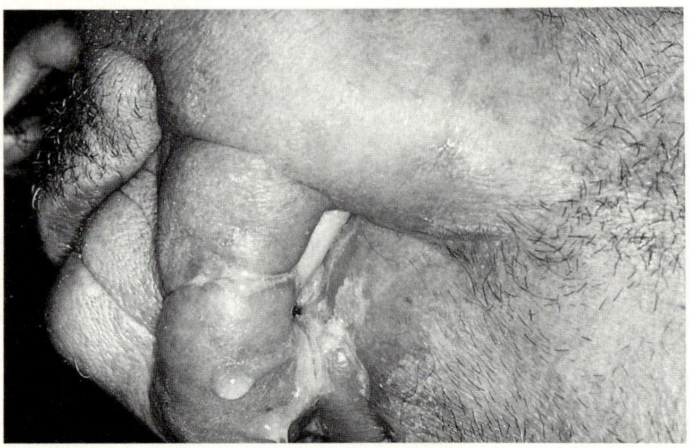

Fig. 2. Clinical photograph demonstrating large orocutaneous fistula with extensive soft tissue loss. The inferior border of the mandible is seen in the center of the orocutaneous fistula. The tissue bed shows other signs of radiation-induced damage, including radiation telangiectasias, severe radiation erythema, and loss of beard growth. Patients with orocutaneous fistulae immediately enter stage 3 protocol

1970s that the introduction of oral bacteria into an essentially avascular bone led to the development of a virulent form of osteomyelitis with extensive hard and soft tissue destruction. The introduction of oral bacteria was felt to be through the trauma of tooth removal, denture wearing, or biopsy. The problem with this concept was that it overlooked the spontaneous cases of osteoradionecrosis of the mandible, as well as the case occurring in the femur, sternum, and clavicle, where obviously no tooth extraction, denture wearing, and frequently no biopsy was taken. Perhaps most importantly, no documentation of culture data or special histologic stains was offered to support this hypothesis. As a follow-up to the inadequacies and lack of scientific substantiation of this hypothesis, Marx (1983a) studied the microbiology of 26 consecutive cases of osteoradionecrosis of the mandible and compared this data to that of bona fide osteomyelitis of the mandible and the long bones. Although many different organisms were consistently identified in all cases of osteomyelitis, no organisms were cultured or observed on histologic sections of the medullary bone of the osteoradionecrotic mandible. As such, Marx (1983a) hypothesized that osteoradionecrosis is a wound-healing problem rather than a primary infection of irradiated bone. Marx (1983a) further elaborated by describing a sequence summarizing the pathophysiology of osteoradionecrosis of the mandible:

1. The administration of tumoricidal radiation therapy
2. The formation of a hypoxic-hypovascular-hypocellular tissue bed
3. Tissue breakdown whereby collagen lysis and cellular death exceed synthesis and cellular replication
4. The development of chronic, nonhealing wounds in which energy, oxygen, and structural precursor demand exceed supply

A review of the radiobiology of osteoradionecrosis of the mandible will further elucidate its pathophysiology.

Radiobiology of Osteoradionecrosis of the Mandible

The goal of radiation therapy is to eradicate the tumor with minimal adverse effects on surrounding normal tissue. A certain degree of residual tissue injury is the understood price for the control of a lethal tumor. The acceptable limits for normal tissue damage vary; however, the integrity and viability of tissues must be maintained whenever possible.

The quantity of radiation delivered to a defined area is the radiation dose, and the time rate at which the dose is administered is the dose rate. Historically, the roentgen and the rad have been units used to describe the measure of radiation dose. The roentgen is defined as a unit of exposure dose for X-rays and gamma rays which produces in $1\,cm^3$ of dry air at standard temperature and pressure ions carrying one electrostatic unit of electricity of either sign. The rad is defined as a unit of absorbed dose and is that amount of radiation of any type that results in the deposition of 100 ergs of energy per g tissue. The new unit gray (Gy) is equivalent to 100 rads. It is the experience of this author and others (Marx and Johnson 1987) that there is a threshold dose of 6000 cGy (60 Gy), independent of surgically or other forms of induced trauma, that may result in spontaneous osteoradionecrosis of the mandible. The amount of soft and hard tissue necrosis, however, is certainly dependent upon the quality and form of radiotherapy. Radiation therapy for head and neck cancer may be delivered as external beam, implant source, neutron beam, or a combination of the above. In a general sense, it has been this author's experience that the most severe cases of tissue destruction are related to implant sources, neutron beam, and higher dose (>7000 cGy) of external beam radiotherapy.

In 1987, Marx and Johnson categorized osteoradionecrosis as either spontaneous or trauma related. Trauma-related cases accounted for 209 (39%) of their reported 536 cases and occurred in a bimodal peak of incidence. The first peak developed in the first 3 months after radiation therapy and was always related to surgical insult either shortly before or during the administration of radiotherapy. In this series, 57 cases were initiated by tooth removal before radiation treatment, ten cases by tooth removal during radiation treatment, and 48 cases by mandibulotomies for access for tumor extirpation followed closely by radiation treatment. The second peak of incidence of trauma-related osteoradionecrosis occurred about 5 years after radiotherapy. These cases may be related to the previously accepted dogma that irradiated tissue gradually recovers with time and to some degree revascularizes. As such, many practitioners had been taught to delay surgical procedures, including tooth removal, in the irradiated mandible for as long as possible to take advantage of this anticipated, but unproven, revascularization. Marx and Johnson (1987) have proved that once more than 6 months have passed, radiotherapy, vascularity, and tissue perfusion progressively decrease and the risk of osteoradionecrosis increases at a nearly arithmetic rate.

The spontaneous form of osteoradionecrosis has been noted to peak about 1 year after radiotherapy and is related to higher doses of external beam therapy, implant source, and a combination of both forms. In general, the radiobiology of osteoradionecrosis is such that the severity of disease is related to increased total dose, increased dose rates (fractions greater than 200 cGy/day), implant sources, neutron beam, concomitant surgery, concomitant chemotherapy, and hyperthermy (Marx and Johnson 1987).

Treatment of Osteoradionecrosis of the Mandible

The treatment of osteoradionecrosis of the mandible in the 1990s is now a time-honored, multifactorial mode of therapy which is based on a staging algorithm (Marx 1983b, 1986). Nonetheless, prior to this protocol, both surgical and nonsurgical methods of treatment had been advocated and still may be performed by many practitioners today. In 1971, Rankow and Weissman recommended treatment of osteoradionecrosis in two stages. Patients were advised to avoid hot and cold foods, smoking, prosthetic appliances, and alcohol. Oral rinses, tetracycline, and analgesics were prescribed. If exposed bone and pain persisted after 1 year or if an orocutaneous fistulae or pathologic fracture developed, the patient would be committed to a mandibular resection.

In 1967, Hahn and Corgill recommended conservative surgical approaches, including drilling holes through the irradiated, nonviable mandibular cortex in order to stimulate granulation tissue. Many of these patients were ultimately committed to continuity resection as well (Marx 1983b). Lengthy courses of antibiotic and analgesic therapy often occurred. Furthermore, multiple, nondefinitive surgical procedures frequently result in greater bone exposure due to the development of nonhealing soft tissue incisions.

In short, the single most important reason that nonsurgical and conservative surgical treatment have failed to cure this disease is that they fail to address the basic pathophysiology of the disease. Furthermore, these nondefinitive forms of therapy have an inherent loss of financial and human resources, as well as the potential for causing drug addictions.

Hyperbaric oxygen has been described (Marx 1983b; Mainous and Hart 1975) as an effective adjunct in the treatment of osteoradionecrosis of the mandible. It was suggested by Hart and Mainous (1976) that the action of hyperbaric oxygen was due to the enhancement of wound healing mediated by vascular proliferation. However, it became clear that hyperbaric oxygen in the absence of aggressive surgical management did not consistently resolve disease. No doubt this was, and continues to be, a result of the great range of presentations and severity of disease. Hyperbaric oxygen's ability to arrest osteoradionecrosis, but not totally resolve it, has led to the Marx surgical–hyperbaric oxygen protocol for the management of osteoradionecrosis (1986). This protocol consists of three stages:

Stage 1. All patients with osteoradionecrosis of the mandible enter stage 1. There are three exceptions to this – patients with pathologic fractures, orocutaneous fistulae, or osteolysis approaching the inferior border of the mandible – who directly enter stage 3. Each stage 1 patient receives 30 hyperbaric oxygen exposures at 2.4 atmospheres absolute pressure (ATA) for 90 min each (at depth) in the multiplace chamber or 2.0 ATA for 120 min (at depth) in the monoplace chamber. All antibiotics are discontinued, and saline rinses may take place. After 30 exposures, the wound is reexamined. If the wound shows improvement such as full mucosal cover, a softening of the bone, or a significant decrease in the size of the exposure, then the patient is labeled a stage 1 responder and completes ten additional hyperbaric oxygen exposures. If no improvement is noted after 30 hyperbaric exposures, then the patient is labeled a stage 1 nonresponder and is advanced to stage 2.

Stage 2. Patients who fail to respond to stage 1 hyperbaric oxygen therapy undergo a marginal alveolar resection of the necrotic bone transorally. If postoperative wound healing occurs, hyperbaric oxygen is continued for only ten additional sessions. If the wound fails to heal, patients are labeled as stage 2 nonresponders and are

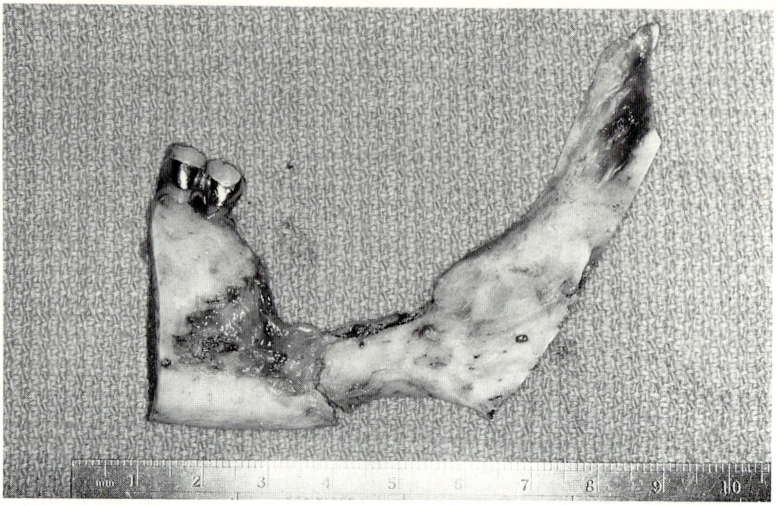

Fig. 3. Specimen from stage 3 continuity resection of osteoradionecrotic mandible. The specimen reveals a previously performed, but unsuccessful, stage 2 marginal resection of the mandible. Removal of the coronoid process with the specimen prevents rotation of the remaining proximal segment and allows for ease in its manipulation during reconstruction of the continuity defect. The presence of fibrous tissue in the fracture site is the attempt of the host, assisted by hyperbaric oxygen therapy, to create a union of the fracture

advanced to stage 3, whereby they are committed to a continuity resection of the affected mandible.

Stage 3. Patients who initially present with a pathologic fracture of the mandible, osteolysis approaching the inferior border of the mandible, or an orocutaneous fistula directly enter stage 3 (Figs. 1, 2). These patients, similar to stage 2 nonresponders, have too much necrotic bone for their disease to respond to anything less than a partial continuity resection of the mandible (Fig. 3). Following 30 sessions of hyperbaric oxygen (40 sessions in the case of stage 2 nonresponders), stage 3 patients undergo a continuity resection of the necrotic mandible back to bleeding margins of bone. The proximal and distal segments may be stabilized with Joe Hall Morris extraskeletal pin fixation. If substantial soft tissue radionecrosis exists, soft tissue reconstruction is performed at the time of mandibular resection. Patients complete ten additional hyperbaric oxygen sessions and advance to stage 3R (reconstruction).

Stage 3R. Reconstruction of the resected osteoradionecrotic mandible is generally performed at least 10 weeks after resection and from a completely transcutaneous approach. This author's commitment to reconstruction of the mandible is just as strong as that of resection of necrotic mandible so as to restore continuity, facial form and function, and frequently the patient's self-esteem.

Prevention of Osteoradionecrosis of the Mandible

The prevention of osteoradionecrosis of the mandible occurs prior to, during, and following tumoricidal radiotherapy. Prior to the administration of tumoricidal radiotherapy, certain surgical procedures with closely followed radiotherapy may predispose the patient to the development of osteoradionecrosis. The first is tooth extraction. Following diagnosis of head and neck cancers, dental practitioners are frequently consulted to remove teeth in the future site of radiotherapy. The second procedure is the mandibulotomy performed in the mandibular angle region for access to tonsillar and base of tongue carcinomas. The mechanism of both involves magnifying tissue injury. Surgical wounding is coupled with radiation wounding, which creates a much greater degree of tissue injury and cellular death than occurs by either factor alone (Marx and Johnson 1987). In these situations, soft and hard tissue does not complete its microscopic, clinical, and radiographic healing, with osteoradionecrosis being the final result. A similar process occurs when teeth are extracted during the administration of radiotherapy.

The prevention of osteoradionecrosis following the administration of radiotherapy is related to the previously mentioned dogma that irradiated tissue recovers with time, which we now understand is not true (Marx and Johnson 1987). Since radiation tissue injury increases with time and hence also increases the probability of the development of osteoradionecrosis, a surgical insult following radiotherapy, with time, may cross the threshold for the development of osteoradionecrosis. The most common surgical insult is tooth extraction in the previously irradiated field.

Prevention of osteoradionecrosis, therefore, begins with the delay of tumoricidal radiotherapy for 21 days following tooth extraction. This, of course, is not possible in many cases of life-threatening cancers, when delay of irradiation may jeopardize the patient's survival. When 21 days cannot pass prior to the administration of radiotherapy, the surgeon, patient, and radiation therapist must understand that a greater risk of osteoradionecrosis exists. The median mandibulotomy as described by SanGiacomo et al. (1992) represents a mechanism to allow for complete cellular healing, since the mandibulotomy is placed out of the irradiated field. The potential for the development of osteoradionecrosis is eliminated, yet adequate surgical access and good cancer principles are achieved in a similar fashion to when a mandibulotomy is performed in the angle region. The extraction of a tooth during the delivery of radiotherapy involves the same detriment to wound healing and, in fact, accounts for the highest risk of osteoradionecrosis (Marx and Johnson 1987). Palliative measures should be taken with teeth identified for removal once radiation has begun. These should continue until radiation has been completed, followed by a course of hyperbaric oxygen therapy to 20 exposures. The teeth may be removed, and ten additional hyperbaric oxygen sessions are delivered postoperatively (Marx et al. 1985). Similarly, anytime after completion of radiation therapy, even years later, surgical procedures in the radiated field should be performed after a similar course of 20 preoperative hyperbaric oxygen sessions, followed by ten postoperative sessions. The angiogenesis that occurs as a result of hyperbaric oxygen therapy allows for a reduction of complications of healing in heavily irradiated tissues (>5000 cGy). As such, prophylactic hyperbaric oxygen therapy should be instituted when surgical procedures are to be performed in an irradiated mandible that has received more than 5000 cGy. In their series of 37 patients undergoing the extraction of 135 teeth in irradiated mandibles (>6000 cGy), Marx et al. (1985) reported an incidence of osteoradionecrosis occurring in 22.9% of the sockets when preoperative hyperbaric oxygen was not administered. This compares to osteoradionecrosis occurring in only 2.6% of 156 extraction sockets in patients who underwent preoperative hyperbaric oxygen therapy. With an inherently better blood supply, a heavily irradiated maxilla is generally able to accomplish uncomplicated wound healing when biopsies of maxillary soft tissues and maxillary teeth are removed in the absence of preoperative hyperbaric oxygen therapy.

Conclusion

Osteoradionecrosis of the mandible is a very debilitating and frequently painful disease process which occurs in a variety of clinical and radiographic presentations. A better understanding of its pathophysiology allows the practitioner to predictably treat patients with this disease and, under ideal circumstances, often prevent its development as well. With the appropriate sequence of treatment, patients may be reconstructed and rehabilitated to enable them to return to the mainstream of life.

References

Ewing J (1926) Radiation osteitis. Acta Radiol 6:399–412

Hahn G, Corgill DA (1967) Conservative treatment of radionecrosis of the mandible. Oral Surg 24:707–711

Happonen RP, Viander M, Pelliniemi L, Aitasalo K (1983) Actinomyces israelii in osteoradionecrosis of the jaws. Histologic and immunocytochemical study of five cases. Oral Surg Oral Med Oral Pathol 55:580–588

Hart GB, Mainous EG (1976) The treatment of radiation necrosis with hyperbaric oxygen. Cancer 37:2580–2585

Mainous EG, Hart GB (1975) Osteoradionecrosis of the mandible: treatment with hyperbaric oxygen. Arch Otolaryngol 101:173–177

Marx RE (1983a) Osteoradionecrosis: a new concept of its pathophysiology. J Oral Maxillofac Surg 41:283–288

Marx RE (1983b) A new concept in the treatment of osteoradionecrosis. J Oral Maxillofac Surg 41:351–357

Marx RE (1986) Hyperbaric oxygen in osteoradionecrosis of the jaw. Infect Surg 348–356

Marx RE, Johnson RP (1987) Studies in the radiobiology of osteoradionecrosis and their clinical significance. Oral Surg Oral Med Oral Pathol 64:379–390

Marx RE, Johnson RP, Kline S (1985) Prevention of osteoradionecrosis: a randomized prospective clinical trial of hyperbaric oxygen versus penicillin. JADA 111:49–54

Meyer I (1970) Infectious diseases of the jaws. J Oral Surg 28:17–26

Obwegeser HL, Sailer HF (1978) Experience with intraoral resection and immediate reconstruction in cases of radio-osteomyelitis of the mandible. J Maxillofac Surg 6:257–265

Phemister DB (1926) Radium necrosis of bone. Am J Roentgenol 16:340–348

Rankow RM, Weissman B (1971) Osteoradionecrosis of the mandible. Ann Otol Rhinol Laryngol 80:603–611

SanGiacomo TR, Goodwin WJ, Stevens MR (1992) Reduction of the median mandibulotomy with the fixed mandibular implant. J Oral Maxillofac Surg 50:292–296

Titterington WP (1971) Osteomyelitis and osteoradionecrosis of the jaws. J Oral Med 26:7–16

Epiprosthetic Rehabilitation: Patient's Acceptance of a Facial Epithesis Following Tumor Surgery

G.F. Duncan

Graphica Sculptura Medica, PO Box 446, Rochester, MN 55903, USA

Introduction

Facial epitheses restore by artificial means the appearance and symmetry of the craniofacial region by duplicating the anatomy removed due to surgery or absent or malformed since birth.

The acceptance of an epithesis is dependent upon the patient's confidence that the epithesis looks good (good cosmetic results) and that the epithesis will not fall off resulting in embarrassment and inconvenience. Patients who seem to be most satisfied with their epitheses tell us that its greatest benefit is that it helps them to feel less conspicuous with friends, family, and strangers.

The epiprosthetic rehabilitation of patients following tumor surgery requires a multidisciplinary approach involving three groups, because the restoration of each patient's future is dependent upon a complex interplay of many different factors. The members of each of these three groups – the medical, dental, and nursing staff; the patient, family members, and friends; and the epiprosthetic rehabilitation team – all have different perceptions of what should be done. Therefore, open, sensitive communication and continuing interaction between these groups maximizes the rehabilitation process.

According to Dr. Arthur Bulbulian (1962)[1], the four main requirements for the success of a facial epithesis are: (1) lifelike appearance, (2) correct and secure method of retention, (3) durability, and (4) tissue compatibility.

Lifelike Appearance. Attaining a lifelike, natural appearance depends upon correctly sculpting the missing or malformed anatomy and using color and surface texture to simulate living tissue.

Correct and Secure Method of Retention. Choosing the best method of retention, i.e., medical adhesives, glasses, magnets, in combination with intraoral obdurators or bone-anchored implants depends upon the patient's lifestyle, age, occupation, and type of disease and defect.

Durability. There is a continual search for better materials and techniques that promote the natural appearance and feel of human tissue, yet maintain their form and color under daily stress.

Tissue Compatibility. The form of the epithesis and method of retention should be designed to work with the underlying muscles and anatomical undercuts. The margins of the epithesis should be designed to utilize existing tissue folds and not irritate the tissue in or around the defect.

Technique of Design and Fabrication

The first step in the design process is obtaining a master cast from an impression made of the patient's defect and contralateral anatomy. Guidelines are drawn using a lipstick pencil to indicate important anatomical landmarks. Impression material backed with plaster bandage is applied to the face. After a short waiting period, the impression is removed from the patient's face. The lipstick guidelines transfer to the master cast. These guidelines, as well as specially marked glasses, enables the medical sculptor/prosthetist to orient the preliminary prototype with consistent accuracy on the patient's face or on the master cast.

The second step is sculpting a natural-looking reproduction of the missing anatomy. The sculpting stage requires looking at patient photos, making preliminary drawings if photos are not available, meeting with friends and family members, listening to the patient's wishes, fears, and expectations, and utilizing all the artistic and anatomical knowledge necessary to create not only the illusion of human tissue, but also human expression.

Patient Acceptance

One of the main features of cancer surgery is the requirement of the surgeon to remove a considerable section of tissue adjacent to the tumor. In many cases, this results in considerable postoperative deformity. The need for psychological adjustment on the part of the patient and the design challenge for the medical sculptor arise from the fact that what was once a familiar face is changed by the resulting surgical defect as well as the epithesis sculpted to fit the defect. The challenge for this patient is looking in the mirror and seeing a new, but unfamiliar face.

Ideal Epiprosthetic Rehabilitation

The ideal surgical preparation of a defect for a facial epithesis can be achieved in the orbital region where: (a) the eyebrow has been preserved to camouflage the superior border of the epithesis, (b) the bony walls of the orbit are contoured and covered with a skin graft, (c) the inferior orbital marginal rim is firm and does not sag due to the weight of the epithesis, and (d) there is adequate depth and height to position the epithesis posteriorly and superiorly. Unfortunately, not all cancer surgery falls into this ideal category. In the management of malignant disease in the maxillofacial region, it is sometimes considered necessary to leave surgically unreconstructed open defects where the maxilla, zygomatic bone, nasal bone, and/or orbital cavity have been removed. In this case, the epithesis bridges the remaining anatomy like a protective bandage: restoring facial symmetry, creating an airway, and helping to reestablish understandable speech by closing off the defect.

Retention Versus Life-style

An epithesis is more readily accepted by the patient when its method of retention fits into the person's life-style. Following tumor surgery, an 83-year-old patient did not want to look in the mirror and see an empty orbit when positioning the epithesis using medical adhesive. Therefore, a family member took over the daily responsibility of applying the glue and positioning the epithesis. However, this did not satisfy the patient psychologically, nor did she want the facial epithesis attached to glasses. When she heard about bone-anchored implants, she practically ran to the operating room. Why? Because she wanted personal control of her appearance. The epithesis is anchored with three magnets and literally pops into proper position. When sneezing or coughing, the patient puts her hand over the epithesis. The majority of patients prefer using medical adhesives to retain their epitheses securely in place. Epitheses are attached to glasses for patients who do not want to have to properly clean and glue the epithesis on every day. Quite often these patients live alone and/or have other physical handicaps. The advantage of retaining the epithesis on the glasses is the obvious ease and convenience as well as air circulation to the underlying tissue. The disadvantage is that when the patient wants to take off the glasses, the defect is exposed.

Durability and Esthetics

Chemists and engineers have sophisticated ways of measuring the shore hardness, the tensile strength, and the elongation of the silicones and urethanes used in the designing of facial epitheses. A patient measures durability by how long an epithesis maintains its life-like appearance. Presently, no synthetic material or pigment is immune to fading. The epitheses start looking "tired." Making repairs and retouching the surface is possible, but extrinsic coloration does not bond as well to a 12-month-old epithesis as to a freshly cured silicone surface.

Facial epitheses are color-matched to the patient's skin using a mixture of the three primary colors, red, blue, and yellow, and usually one or two additional colors such as burnt or raw umber, yellow ocher, or emerald green. This creates the so-called intrinsic base color. Depending on the type of silicone and individual working methods, one can paint capillaries, shadows under the eyes, freckles, etc., directly onto the mold surface.

With proper care and maintenance, a silicone epithesis lasts between 6 months and 2 years. Silicone is a synthetic material. The thin margins tear and the color changes. The daily application and removal of medical adhesive increases the incidence of torn thin margins to a greater extent than with bone-anchored epitheses or epitheses attached to glasses.

Tissue Compatibility

The form of the epithesis and all methods of retention should be designed to work with the movement of the underlying muscles and anatomical undercuts as well as to provide protection for the defect, preventing the entrance of foreign objects into the open defect. Beginning with the wax/clay prototype, the margins should be contoured to utilize existing tissue and not irritate the tissue in or around the defect.

Conclusion

Social compatibility as well as tissue compatibility have to be taken into consideration. People like social contact and social acceptance. Even for a blind person, who does not have to suffer the stares and questioning looks from friends and family, it is important to feel "whole." Sensitive listening and communication with the patient is an important part of the rehabilitation process. A facial epithesis should be a morale builder – providing the patient with a sense of self-confidence and predictability about how they perceive themselves as well as how others see them.

Reference

Bulbulian A (1962) Modern facial prosthetics. Med Biol Illustration VII 2:92–97

Value of Follow-Up in Patients Treated for Squamous Cell Carcinomas of the Oral Cavity and Oropharynx

M. Boysen

Department of Otolaryngology, National Hospital, University of Oslo, 0027 Oslo, Norway

Introduction

The follow-up of patients with head and neck carcinomas may be conducted for a variety of reasons, including assessing the efficiency of treatment and its morbidity, providing psychological and social support, and evaluating treatment results. The main purpose, however, is to detect relapse at a stage at which effective secondary treatment can be given. Regular attendance is costly and makes up a major part of the workload of many outpatient clinics. It is, therefore, important that the effectiveness of the detection of relapse and the influence this has on the patient's subsequent clinical course are evaluated. The value of follow-up has been questioned for several types of carcinomas, including head and neck carcinomas (Boysen et al. 1985; Bröyn and Fröyen 1982; Cochrane et al. 1980; Eckman et al. 1977; Wolfsenberger 1988).

This report, which is part of a larger prospective series of patients with head and neck carcinomas (Boysen et al. 1992), focuses on the efficiency of long-term follow-up of oral and oropharyngeal carcinomas in detecting relapses and second malignant tumors.

Material and Methods

During the 5-year period from May 1983 to May 1988, 364 previously untreated patients with confirmed squamous cell carcinoma of the oral cavity and oropharynx were consecutively admitted to our department. Clinical findings, treatment, results, and outcome of all follow-up consultations were recorded prospectively. Excluded from the present study were 21 patients with disseminated disease, other serious illnesses, or poor general condition which would have made treatment with curative intent impossible. Furthermore, 62 patients in whom initial control of the primary tumor and/or neck metastases was not achieved were also excluded (i.e., patients where the operative findings or histological examination of the surgical specimens showed an incomplete resection and patients who had residual tumor locally, regionally, or at distant sites at the first follow-up visit 6 weeks after completion of the treatment). This left 281 patients who were considered free of disease 6 weeks after the completion of treatment. Their average age was 64 years (range, 27–87 years), and two thirds of the patients were males. The Union International Contra le Cancrum (UICC) classification of 1982 (Harmer 1982) was used to stage the tumors.

In general, the smaller tumors (T1–2) were given radiotherapy with surgery for suspected residual tumor, and the larger, planned preoperative radiotherapy and surgery whenever possible. In cases where resection of a part of the mandible was considered necessary, surgery usually preceded radiotherapy. Radiotherapy was given in once-daily fractions of 2 Gy 5 days a week (some patients received 2.35 Gy 4 days a week) from an external megavolt source directed towards the primary site and usually both sides of the entire neck. The primary site received 66–80 Gy. Most cases of oral carcinomas not involving the mandible received external irradiation of 47–50 Gy and an additional 20–30 Gy as brachytherapy for the primary tumor. The clinically negative neck received 47–50 Gy and the positive neck an additional boost of 10 Gy to the nodes followed by neck dissection.

Follow-up data consisted of the number of clinical visits, the data and site of relapse, and the result of the secondary treatment. Also recorded were the way relapses were detected: (a) by symptoms or signs that the patients reported at the scheduled (routine) follow-up visits or interval visits requested by the patients or (b) through physical examination alone at routine visits. For second malignancies, the criteria proposed by Warren and Gates (1932) were applied. Carcinomas of the skin were not included.

In general, the patients were seen at the outpatient clinic at 2- to 3-month intervals during the first 2 years, every 3–4 months during the following 3 years, and twice a year thereafter. The consultations included general ear, nose, and throat (ENT) examination supplemented with endoscopic examination, when indicated, and relevant blood tests. X-ray of the chest and panendoscopy (hypopharyngo-, oesophagoscopy-, laryngo-, and bronchoscopy) were not routinely included in the work-up. None of the patients were lost to follow-up, and the minimum duration of follow-up was 3.5 years. Death certificates were obtained for deceased patients, and autopsy records were reviewed when available. The results were analyzed as of 1 December 1991.

The SAS (Statistical Analysis System) 6.03 software for personal computers (SAS Institute Inc., Cary, NC, USA) was used for the storage and processing of the data. The Kaplan-Meier method was used to determine the actuarial risk of developing second malignant tumors (Matthews and Farewell 1988).

Results

Almost half the patients had stage III or IV disease (Table 1) and a total of 95 patients (34%) developed relapse; Table 2 reveals the distribution of the first relapse according to the site of the primary tumor. Almost half the relapses were detected during the first year (Fig. 1) and 14 (15%) after the third year of initiation of treatment. The distribution of the site of recurrences was equal for all time periods.

In 58% (55/95), the patients themselves had noticed symptoms or signs such as pain, soreness, increased hoarseness, or a lump in the neck suggesting some irregularity that eventually led to the diagnosis of relapse. Particularly symptoms and signs suggesting a regional recurrence were often noticed by the patients (19/22). Forty patients (42%) with relapse had no

Table 1. Clinical classification (Harmer 1982) according to the site of the primary tumor

Site of primary tumor	Classification		
	Stage I+II	Stage III+IV	All
Oral cavity			
Floor of mouth	35	15	50
Tongue	54	30	84
Alveolar process, buccal, hard palate	37	39	76
All	126	84	210
Oropharyngeal			
Tonsillar	11	32	43
Base of tongue	3	11	14
Posterior wall, soft palate	7	7	14
All	21	50	71
Total	147	134	281

Table 2. Number and site of first relapses according to the site of the primary tumor

Site of relapse	Site of primary tumor		
	Oral cavity (n = 210)	Oro-pharyngeal (n = 71)	Total (n = 281)
Local	49	9	58 (21%)
Regional	21	1	22 (8%)
Distant	5	10	15 (5%)
Total	75 (36%)	20 (28%)	95 (34%)

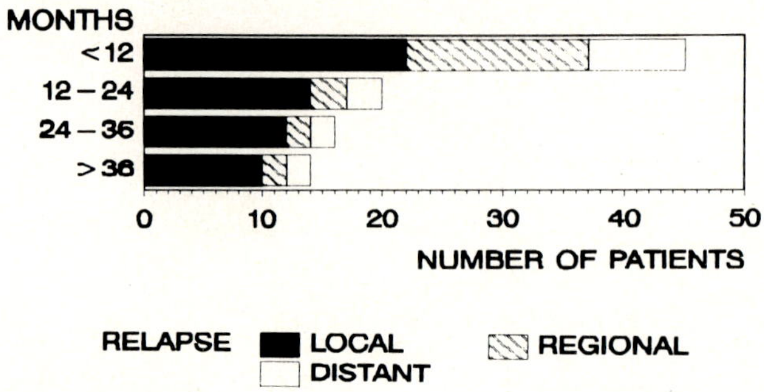

Fig. 1. Site of relapse and time from initiation of treatment to diagnosis of relapse

Table 3. How the first relapse was detected

Means of detection	Site of relapse			
	Local	Regional	Distant	Total
Symptoms presented by the patient	30	19	6	55 (58%)
Physical examination	28	3	9	40 (42%)
Total	58	22	15	95 (100%)

Table 4. Status following first relapse according to stage in patients with oral carcinomas

Status	Stage and site of relapse						
	Stage I+II			Stage III+IV			All
	Local	Regional	Distant	Local	Regional	Distant	
ANED	10	0	0	1	0	1	12
DOD	5	2	0	0	1	0	8
DFD	14	11	1	19	7	3	55
	29	13	1	20	8	4	75

ANED, alive, no evidence of disease; DOD, dead from other disease; DFD, dead from disease.

apparent symptoms, and the relapse was diagnosed by physical examination alone at the scheduled follow-up visits (Table 3).

None of the 20 patients with relapse of oropharyngeal carcinomas were salvaged through additional treatment. Table 4 shows the result of secondary treatment in patients with oral carcinomas. Secondary treatment of local relapse proved efficient almost exclusively in patients with stage I and II

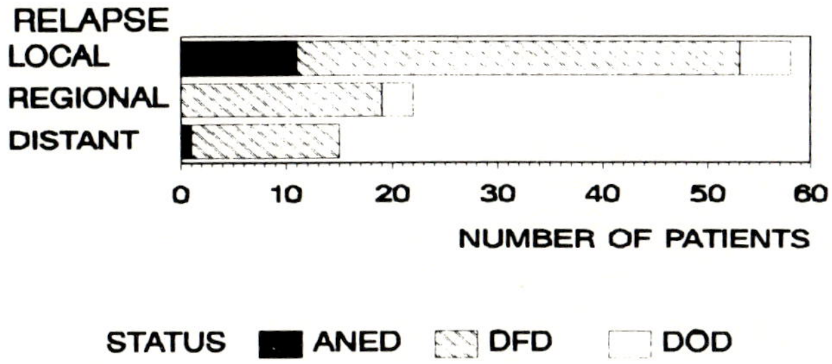

Fig. 2. Results of relapse treatment (*ANED*, alive no evidence of disease; *DFD*, dead from disease; *DOD*, dead other diseases)

Table 5. Number of routine follow-up visits, first relapses, and cures according to the year of follow-up

	Year following initiation of treatment 1	2	3	>4	Total
No. of follow-up visits	1043	753	629	516	2941
No. of relapses	45	20	16	14	95
("relapse pick-up rate")	1/23	1/38	1/39	1/36	1/31
No. of cured patients	7	3	5	5	20
("relapse cure rate")	1/149	1/251	1/126	1/103	1/147
("follow-up cure rate")[1]	6.4	6.7	3.2	2.8	4.8

[1] Relationship between number of relapses and number of cures.

tumors – all had initially been treated with radiotherapy alone or radiotherapy combined with limited resections. Only one patient with an advanced tumor (T3) was salvaged. Of the 21 patients with regional recurrences of oral carcinomas, none are still alive: 14 had received treatment with curative intent; three patients (14%), all with previously untreated necks, died from other diseases without evidence of disease in the neck; and an additional two patients died from distant relapse without evidence of remaining disease in the neck. One of the 15 patients with distant relapse was cured. Figure 2 summarizes the results of relapse treatment.

The 281 patients made a total of 3589 follow-up visits. Of these, 2941 were follow-up visits prior to the first relapse, death from other diseases, or last regular follow-up visit. The "relapse pick-up rate" (number of visits necessary to diagnose one relapse) was approximately the same for all time periods (Table 5). During the first year of follow-up, relapses were more frequently detected through physical examination than through symptoms and signs being noticed by the patient. Later on, the opposite was the case, and after the third year only one of 14 relapses were detected through

Table 6. Number and site of second malignant tumors and how they were diagnosed

Means of detection	Site second malignant tumor				Total
	Head & neck	Lung	Esophagus	Other	
Symptoms presented by the patient	16	8	9	7	40 (85%)
Physical examination	5	2	0	0	7 (15%)
Total	21 (45%)	10 (21%)	9 (19%)	7 (15%)	47 (100%)

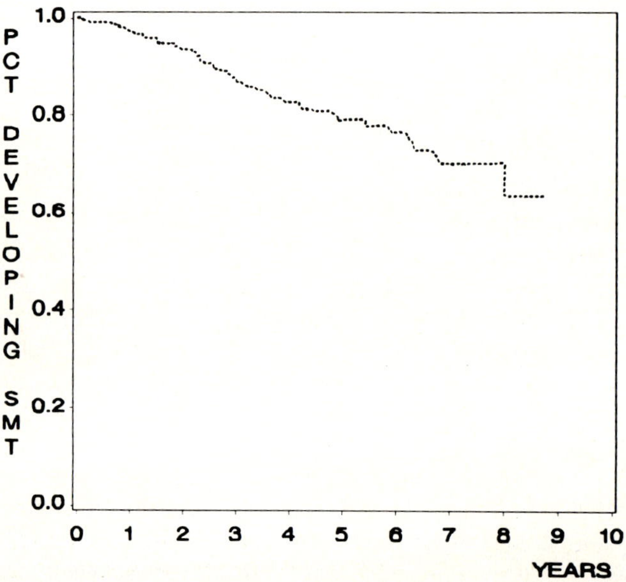

Fig. 3. The Kaplan-Meier estimated incidence of second malignant tumors (*SMT*) in patients (*PCT*) with index tumor in the oral cavity and oropharynx

physical examination. In addition, the number of cures in relation to the number of follow-up visits ("relapse cure rate") was almost equal for all time periods. On the other hand, the "follow-up cure rate" (number of cures in relation to the number of relapses) decreased with the time the patients were followed (Table 5).

Patients with oral stage I and II disease made a total of 1320 (45%) follow-up visits during the first 3 years of follow-up. The remaining 1621 visits (55%) were made after the third year by patients with oropharyngeal tumors and for advanced stages of oral carcinomas. For this latter group, two patients (one local and one distant relapse) are alive and one died from intercurrent disease.

A total of 47 patients (17%) developed second malignant tumors (Table 6); seven (15%) of these (five within the head and neck region and two lung carcinomas) were diagnosed through clinical examination at scheduled visits. In the remaining 85%, the diagnosis was obtained through symptoms or signs presented by the patients which led to further examination either in our department, through consultation with a private physician, or at the local hospital. Second malignant tumors developed at a relatively constant rate of approximately 4% per year (Fig. 3). Fifteen patients were alive when the study was closed; ten of these had second malignancies in the head and neck region and three had lung carcinomas. Second malignant tumors accounted for 16% of deaths.

Discussion

Routine follow-up of patients considered to be curatively treated for carcinoma has several objectives, the main purpose being early detection and treatment of relapse. Regular follow-up visits are also performed in order to register and treat complications that treatment may have caused, to provide help in relieving psychosocial and physical problems, to detect and treat second neoplasms, and finally to evaluate results and report end points.

The search for relapse of carcinoma at routine follow-up visits presupposes that new manifestations of the disease are more likely to be cured if detected at the earliest possible moment. Studies concerning cancer of the breast (Bröyn et al. 1982; Dewar and Kerr 1985), colon (Cochrane et al. 1980; Ekman et al. 1977), bronchial carcinoma (Kolb and Buchman 1985), and a large regional follow-up program covering several types of carcinomas (Queisser et al. 1990) all suggest that routine follow-up was of limited benefit in terms of increased survival. Similar studies on patients with head and neck carcinomas indicate that follow-up is only meaningful for patients for whom there are treatment options left, and even then only for a certain period of time (Boysen et al. 1985, 1992; Wolfensberger 1988).

Successful treatment of relapse was almost exclusively achieved in local recurrences of relative small (T1 and T2) oral carcinomas treated with radiotherapy alone or where radiotherapy was combined with limited resections. Independent of the initial treatment, the results of secondary treatment of local relapse of advanced local disease were disappointing. Likewise, the results of regional recurrences in previously treated necks, both those receiving elective treatment (mostly radiotherapy) and N-positive necks, were discouraging. Only three of the 22 regional relapses were apparently cured, all of these in patients with previously untreated necks. At the end of the study, however, they had all died as a result of intercurrent diseases. An additional two patients receiving secondary treatment of regional relapse died from distant metastases without evidence of renewed tumor growth in the neck.

The surprisingly low regional relapse pick-up rate may be the consequence of our follow-up regime allowing too few visits during the first 2–3 years of follow-up (Snow 1992). The inability to detect early regional relapses may to some extent be explained by changes in the soft tissue induced by high-dose radiotherapy. Due to these changes, early detection of regional relapses through palpation alone may be impossible. Recent investigations using ultrasound for detection of neck nodes and ultrasound-guided aspiration cytology have proved very effective in detecting tumor-positive nodes in the initial work-up (van Brekel et al. 1991; Baatenburg de Jough et al. 1989). Whether this method is also useful in detecting early regional relapses is not known at present and should be subjected to further evaluation.

The number of relapses decreased with time, and only 15% occurred after the third year following initiation of treatment. In spite of decreasing frequency of follow-up visits with the time the patients were followed, the proportion of cures in relation to the number of relapses remained approximately the same. This observation, together with the fact that a decreasing number of relapses were detected through clinical examination, suggests that late relapses do not do worse than early ones. Furthermore, if we take into consideration the fact that the follow-up cure rate decreased with the time the patients were followed and that late relapses were almost exclusively detected through symptoms presented by the patients, one may raise the question as to whether regular follow-up visits designed to detect relapses are indeed required after the third year of follow-up. In spite of improved diagnostic tools such as computed tomography (CT), magnetic resonance imaging (MRI), and possibly ultrasound-guided aspiration cytology, it is likely that providing detailed information for patients about the symptoms and signs that may occur and encouraging them to contact our outpatient clinic as soon as alarming symptoms arise may prove to be as important in detecting early relapse as regular follow-up

The majority of our patients have undergone high-dose radiotherapy and/or mutilating operations. It is the responsibility of the institutions treating these patients to initiate and maintain the necessary functional adjustment and substitutional therapy. Furthermore, many patients may need psychological, social, and occupationally related rehabilitation. Long-term follow-up is often necessary to cope with all kinds of rehabilitation. However, these consultations need not be on a regular basis, but can be tailored to meet individual needs.

Second malignant tumors following carcinomas of the head and neck occur at a rate of 3%–6% a year (Cooper et al. 1989; Tepperman and Fritzpatrick 1981; Vikram et al. 1984). After the third year following completion of the primary detection and treatment, these tumors become a cause of greater concern than relapses. Surprisingly, only 15% of the second malignant neoplasma were detected through clinical examinations, suggesting that our follow-up in this respect was insufficient. It should be noted that neither regular panendoscopic examination nor chest X-ray was part of our follow-up program. Bronchoscopy may detect a significant number of second malignancies in the lungs (Leipzig et al. 1985; McGuirt 1982). Even in early stages, patients with these tumors have poor survival rates (Atabeck et al. 1987; Shons and McQuarrie 1985). In the present material, ten patients developed second malignancies in the lungs; however, it is questionable whether the costs and effort connected with regular bronchoscopy could improve the survival rate to such an extent as to justify them (Shaha et al. 1988).

If the sole purpose of follow-up is detection of recurrences, regular follow-up may largely be omitted for patients with oropharyngeal carcinomas and advanced stages of oral carcinomas. In addition, follow-up visits beyond the third year after the initiation of treatment were of little value in terms of increased survival. The follow-up in these patients should mainly be to provide care and support and can be carried out on an individual basis. A part of the work-load saved by excluding unnecessary visits could be redirected to intensify the follow-up during the first 2–3 years for patients for whom treatment options are still open. In any case, the number of follow-up visits could be reduced by approximately one third without reducing the care and support that we are obliged to give. The means, personnel, and time thus made available could be better utilized.

Acknowledgement. This study was supported by the Norwegian Cancer Society.

References

Atabek U, Mohit-Tabatabai MA, Raina S, Rush BF, Dasmahapatra KS (1987) Lung cancer in patients with head and neck cancer. Incidence and long-term survival. Am J Surg 154:434–438

Baatenburg de Jongh RJ, Rongen RJ, Lameris JS, Harthoorn M, Vervoerd CDA, Knegt P (1989) Metastatic neck disease: palpation vs. ultrasound examination. Arch Otolaryngol Head Neck Surg 115:689–690

Boysen M, Natvig K, Winther FÖ, Tausjö J (1985) Value of routine follow-up in patients treated for squamous cell carcinoma of the head and neck. J Otolaryngol 14:211–214

Boysen M, Løvdal O, Tausjø J, Winther F (1992) The value of follow-up in patients treated for squamous cell carcinoma of the head and neck. Eur J Cancer 28: 426–430

Bröyn T, Fröyen J (1982) Evaluation of routine follow-up after surgery for breast carcinoma. Acta Chir Scand 148:401–404

Cochrane JPS, Williams JT, Faber RG, Slack WW (1980) Value of outpatient follow-up after curative surgery for carcinoma of the large bowel. Br Med J 280:593–595

Cooper JS, Pajak TF, Rubin P, Tuppchong L, Brady LW, Leibel SA, Laramore GE, Marcial VA, Davis LW, Cox JD (1989) Second malignancies in patients who have head and neck cancer: incidence, effect on survival and implications based on the RTOG experience. Int J Radiat Oncol Biol Phys 17:449–456

Dewar JR, Kerr GR (1985) Value of routine follow-up of women treated for early carcinoma of the breast. Br Med J 291:1464–1467

Ekman C-A, Gustavson J, Henning A (1977) Value of follow-up study of recurrent carcinoma of the colon and rectum. Surg Gynecol Obstet 145:895–897

Harmer MH (ed) (1982) Classification of malignant tumors, 3rd edn. UICC, Geneva 1987 (revised 1982)

Kolb E, Buchmann P (1985) Erfahrungen bei Langzeitenuntersuchungen von Patienten mit radikal operiertem Bronchuskarzinom. Schweiz Rundschau Med (Praxis) 74:1017–1020

Leipzig B, Zellmer JE, Klug D et al. (1985) The role of endoscopy in evaluating patients with head and neck cancer: a multi-institutional prospective study. Arch Otolaryngol 111:589–594

Matthews DE, Farewell VT (eds) (1988) Using and understanding medical statistics. Karger, Basel, pp 67–78

McGuirt WF (1982) Panendoscopy as a screening examination for simultaneous primary tumors in head and neck cancer: a prospective sequential study and review of the literature. Laryngoscope 92:569–576

Neel HB (1984) Routine endoscopy – is it necessary every time. Arch Otolaryngol 110:531–532

Queisser W, Maurer U, Schmidt H (1990) Efficacy of German regional follow-up program of 5411 cancer patients. J Cancer Res Clin Oncol 116 Suppl 1:206

Schuller DE, Fritsch MH (1986) An assessment of the value of triple endoscopy in the evaluation of head and neck cancer patients. J Surg Oncol 32:156–158

Shaha A, Hoover E, Marti J, Krespi Y (1988) Is routine triple endoscopy cost-effective in head and neck cancer? Am J Surg 155:750–753

Shons AR, McQuarrie DG (1985) Multiple primary epidermoid carcinomas of the upper aerodigestive tract. Arch Surg 120:1007–1009

Snow GB (1992) Follow-up in patients treated for head and neck cancer: how frequent, how thorough and for how long? Eur J Cancer 28:315–316

Tepperman BS, Fitzpatrick PJ (1981) Second respiratory and upper digestive tract cancer after oral cancer. Lancet ii:547–549

van den Brekel JWM, Castelijns JA, Stel HV, Luth WJ, Valk J, Waal van der I, Snow GB (1991) Occult metastatic neck disease: detection with US and US-guided fine needle aspiration cytology. Radiology 180:457–461

Vikram B, Strong ES, Shah JP, Spiro R (1984) Second malignant neoplasms in patients successfully treated with multimodality treatment for advanced head and neck cancer. Head Neck Surg 6:734–737

Warren S, Gates O (1932) Multiple primary malignant tumors: a survey of literature and statistical study. Am J Cancer 16:1358–1414

Wolfensberger M (1988) Aufwand und Nutzen regelmässiger Nachkontrollen bei Patienten mit Plasterzellkarzinomen des Larynx, der Mundhöhle und des Pharynx. HNO 36:28–32

Subject Index

Anastomosis 27
Angiogenesis 198
Anterior cranial fossa 18
Atmospheres absolute pressure
(ATA) 195

Benign tumors 30
Bleomycin 135
Buthionine sulfoximine 187

Cancer 4
oral cavity 4
oropharynx 4
tonsil 140
Candida albicans 14
Carboplatin 89, 140
Carboplatin in vitro 97
Carcinogenesis 183
Carcinoma
floor of Mouth 101
oropharynx 112, 145
tongue 101, 140
Carcinoma in situ 11
Cavernous sinus 20
Cell kinetics 116
Cervical lymph nodes metastases 44
Cisplatin 89, 135, 137, 166, 187
Clinically negative neck 81
Clinically positive neck 83
Clival involvement 20
Complication rates 139
Computed tomography 44
Curietherapy 101

Design and fabrication 202
DNA ploidy 93
DÖSAK Study 157
Drug Resistance 186
Durability and Esthetics 203

Elective neck treatment 82
Epidemiological studies
interventional 7
prospective 155
prospective cohort 7
retrospective case-control studies 7
Epidemiology of cancer 1
Epiprosthetic rehabilitation 201
Epithelial dysplasia 9, 11, 14
Erythroplakia 9, 10, 15
Excisional or incisional biopsy 85
Extended Anterior Resection 22
External Irradiation 101

Facial epithesis 201
Facial esthetics 25
"Fingerprints" 12
Follow-up 205
Free autogenous bone 30
Free jejunal grafts 27, 40
Frozen section analysis 21
5c ratio 94
5-FU 96

Gray (Gy) 137, 193

Head and Neck carcinoma 111, 170
Head and Neck contracts
programm 135
Hemiglossectomy 26
Hyperbaric oxygen 195

Hyperfractionated and Accelerated Irradiation 66
Hyperfractionation 96, 111

Immunotherapy 184
Implants 30, 31
Incidence 3
Induction chemotherapy 65, 133
Interleukin-2 (IL-2) 185
Irradiation 30

Laryngeal cancer 138
Larynx 137
Lateral rhinotomy 19
Leucoplakia 9, 10, 12, 14
Local transposition flaps 26
Locoregional control 112, 147

Magnetic resonance imaging 45
Malignant tumors 31
Mandibulotomy 197
Maxillary sinus carcinoma 17
Maxillofacial tumors 25
Metastases, distant 135, 141
  regional 138
Methotrexat 135
Micronucleus formation 93
Microvascular bone grafting 29
Microvascular surgery 27
Mitoguazone 139
Monoclonal antibodies (mab) 186
Morbidity of treatment 135
Multicenter DÖSAK study 155
Myocutaneous flap 40
Myofacial flap 40

National survey 23
Neck dissection 85
  conservative 59
  elective 48
  radikal 59
  terminology 57
  therapeutic 50
Nitrosamines 15

Organ preservation 137
Oropharyngeal carcinoma 112
Osteoradionecrosis 191
  mandible 191
  non healing wounds 193

Patient acceptance 202
Population-based cancer registers 3
Precancerous condition 9
Precancerous lesions 9
Prevalence of leucoplakia 11
Prevention 183
Primary prevention 1
Prognostic factors 43

Radiation Therapy Oncology Group (RTOG) 145
Radiochemotherapy 89, 166
  combined 66
  preoperative 156, 165
Radiosensitizer 65
Radiotherapy 34, 63, 166, 197, 206
  accelerated 111
  accelerated superfractionation 76
  acute and late tolerance 112
  acute toxicity 76
  hyperfractionated 111, 145
  hyperfractionated and accelerated 94
  noncomitant boost irradiation 71
  once daily 69
  postoperative 51
  preoperative 156, 165
  twice daily 69, 84
Radiotherapy and simultaneous cisplatin 170
Recurrence 207
Relapse pick-up rate 209
Results 205
Results of secondary treatment 211
Retention 203
Retinoid receptors 184
Risk factors 7

Secondary treatment 208
Second malignancies 206
Second malignant tumors 211
Second primary tumors 121
Skull base 23
Skull base surgery 18
Snuff-induced lesions 12
Soft tissue radionecrosis 196
Speech ability 29
Speech results 29
Squamous Cell 101
Squamous Cell carcinoma 11, 101, 133, 165
  oral cavity 69, 166, 205
    floor of the mouth 101
    pharynx 133
    tongue 101
Subclinical disease 83
Sulfhydryls 187
Superfractionated and accelerated irradiation 69

Surgery 206
  interposed 92
  radical 155
Surgery for malignant disease 23
Surgery of oropharyngeal cancer 37
Surgical management of cervical
  lymph nodes 43
Survival 73

Tissue compatibility 204
Tobacco consumption 7, 12
Treatment 205, 207, 211
  of relapse 211
Treatment-dependent prognostic index
  (TPI) 155

Tumor control 73
Tumor infiltrating lymphocytes
  (TIL) 185
Tumor repopulation 91
Tumor volume 70
  analyses 77

Ultrasound 46

Veteran's Affairs Laryngeal Cancer
  Study Group 138
Vitamin A 184
Volume reconstruction 77

Springer-Verlag and the Environment

We at Springer-Verlag firmly believe that an international science publisher has a special obligation to the environment, and our corporate policies consistently reflect this conviction.

We also expect our business partners – paper mills, printers, packaging manufacturers, etc. – to commit themselves to using environmentally friendly materials and production processes.

The paper in this book is made from low- or no-chlorine pulp and is acid free, in conformance with international standards for paper permanency.

Druck: Saladruck, Berlin
Verarbeitung: Buchbinderei Lüderitz & Bauer, Berlin